Stacking Therapies for Depression Recovery

A Layered Healing Approach

Greg Doney

Paperback ISBN: 978-1-7646377-0-1

Hardcover ISBN: 978-1-7646377-1-8

Epub ISBN: 978-1-7646377-2-5

Medical Disclaimer

This book and its contents are provided for informational purposes only. The author and publisher make no representations or warranties regarding the accuracy, completeness, or applicability of the content. They disclaim all liability for any errors, omissions, or inconsistencies that may be present.

The content in this book is not intended to diagnose, treat, cure, or prevent any condition or disease. It is not a substitute for professional medical advice, diagnosis, or treatment. Always consult a licensed healthcare professional before making any changes to your health regimen or treatment plan. The use of this book implies your understanding and acceptance of this disclaimer.

The author and publisher do not guarantee any specific outcomes or results from following the advice or strategies in this book. Individual results will vary, and the examples or testimonials provided are not intended to guarantee similar experiences.

This book does not constitute advice to start, stop, reduce, or change any medication or prescribed treatment. Never alter or discontinue any medication without first consulting your prescribing doctor or psychiatrist.

By reading this book, you accept full responsibility for your health and well-being and agree that the author and publisher are not liable for any decisions or actions you take based on its content.

Contents

The Power of Layered Healing – Building Towards a Brighter Future

A Message of Hope

If you're reading this, it may be because the weight of depression feels overwhelming, making the idea of change seem out of reach. You're not alone in feeling this way. Recovery can often feel daunting, especially when you've tried many things that haven't seemed to help. But here's an empowering truth: there are still options – many options – and this book is here to help you uncover them, one layer at a time.

Small, manageable steps, taken consistently, can create a foundation for real, lasting change. Layered healing is about combining these steps in a supportive, cumulative approach that steadily builds toward relief, strength, and, ultimately, hope. Even small improvements, when stacked together over time, have the potential to change the course of your life and open up new possibilities.

Setting the Goal of Remission

For those with depression, achieving relief – reaching remission – might feel like an ambitious goal, but it is possible.

Remission means experiencing symptom relief and rediscovering a sense of stability and engagement in daily life. This goal of remission is both valuable and achievable, and this book is dedicated to guiding you there.

Beyond remission, it's also possible to continue building layers that improve resilience, deepen health, and enrich your quality of life. These additional "gravy" layers are entirely up to you. Reaching remission alone is powerful and meaningful, and this book is here to support you, whether your goal is remission, long-term strength, or exploring those extra layers that make life feel even brighter.

The Concept of Layered Healing: Building Change, One Step at a Time

Layered healing is about making recovery feel accessible by focusing on small, research-backed changes that add up over time. Imagine this process as stacking improvements, one on top of another, so that each small step has a cumulative effect. Each therapy, lifestyle change, and mindset shift contributes its own benefit to mood, resilience, and mental clarity.

Small improvements have their own unique power; they create momentum, which in turn fuels motivation. For instance, incorporating regular movement has been shown to relieve mood symptoms (Schuch et al., 2016), while improving sleep can lead to a meaningful boost in mental health (Irwin, 2015). Adding nutritious, mood-supporting foods brings additional improvement (Firth et al., 2020). When these changes are layered together, they amplify one another, and what may have felt impossible becomes achievable.

Layered healing takes advantage of this stacking effect, where each layer of healing builds upon the previous ones, creating a powerful, self-sustaining cycle of improvement. Here's how it works:

Individual steps toward relief: Each therapy or lifestyle habit brings its own improvement, even if it seems small. Every step counts and builds your resilience one layer at a time.

Progress that builds on itself: With each new step, previous improvements are reinforced, creating a more lasting, sustainable effect. This is why small changes matter – they build a foundation for continued success, helping each step feel achievable.

Supported by evidence: Every recommendation in this book is backed by research, providing a foundation of scientific support. This approach aligns with international clinical guidelines: the World Federation of Societies for Biological Psychiatry (WFSBP) and the Australasian Society of Lifestyle Medicine (ASLM) position physical activity, sleep, and mindfulness as high-evidence interventions for Major Depressive Disorder. The Royal Australian and New Zealand College of Psychiatrists (RANZCP) uses a biopsychosocial lifestyle (BPSL) model that makes lifestyle interventions a primary clinical recommendation. References are included at the end of each chapter, allowing you to explore the evidence behind each recommendation.

Taking Small Steps That Add Up to Big Change

The process of layered healing encourages you to start wherever you are, with the steps that feel most achievable. Each chapter in this book guides you through practical, evidence-based steps you can take at your own pace. Rather than requiring an immediate overhaul, this approach lets you add layers slowly, helping you with real, achievable actions that build a foundation of well-being.

For example:

Incorporating exercise: Even a 15-minute walk each day can have a significant impact on mood, and over time, can help you feel more empowered and connected to your body.

Improving sleep: Establishing a consistent sleep routine, even just going to bed 15 minutes earlier, can greatly affect mental clarity and energy.

Nourishing your body: Adding one nutritious, mood-supporting meal or snack each day can improve your energy and stabilise mood, providing a reliable source of support.

These small shifts accumulate, creating a ripple effect of healing that goes beyond any single action. The combined approach is powerful precisely because it recognises that incremental change can be both sustainable and transformative.

The Lifespan Impact of Mental Health

Addressing mental health doesn't just improve daily well-being; it supports physical health, longevity, and quality of life. Left untreated, depression and other mental health challenges can impact physical health, increasing the risk for chronic conditions and even reducing life expectancy. Chronic stress, compounded by lifestyle impacts, can contribute to inflammation, lower immune response, and other health risks over time. However, the power of healing lies in reversing this trajectory.

By actively engaging in layered healing and working toward remission, you are not only lifting your mental health but also supporting a longer, healthier life. Small, positive changes – like better sleep, balanced nutrition, and regular movement – affect both mind and body. Layered healing is a proactive path that helps you to reclaim your life, creating a strong foundation for lasting wellness and strength.

The Ripple Effect: Amplifying Your Impact

One of the most empowering aspects of layered healing is that, as you strengthen your own mental health, you may also positively affect those around you. Small changes in self-care, mindset, and strength often ripple outward, inspiring and supporting family, friends, and communities. When you prioritise your health, you create a model of stability that others can see, which can foster a culture of care and empathy in your personal relationships.

Healing can feel isolating, but as you progress, you may find that others are drawn to your journey, encouraged by the strength you've built. Each step you take amplifies this positive effect, helping you and those around you feel more hopeful, connected, and supported.

Summary of Core Principles in Layered Healing

As you move forward with this book, here are a few guiding principles to remember:

Every step counts: No matter how small a change may feel, it adds to the cumulative effect of healing. Trust in the power of incremental progress.

Build slowly, sustainably: Layered healing is about sustainable change. Take each chapter and step at your own pace, allowing each new layer to settle before moving forward.

Celebrate each milestone: Healing is a process with many small victories. Each improvement – no matter how slight – brings you closer to your goal.

Resilience grows over time: Every layer strengthens the foundation of your recovery, making each improvement feel a bit more stable, a bit more achievable. Over time, these layers create strength, making it easier to face life's challenges.

Moving Forward: The Next Steps in Your Journey

Your path forward doesn't need to be set in stone. Layered healing is flexible, adaptable to your needs, and designed to evolve with you. Each layer provides a foundation for the next, helping you reach a brighter future with small, achievable steps. Remember that healing is not just about getting better – it's about building a life that feels meaningful, strong, and fulfilling.

Continue your process with patience, celebrate each small step, and embrace the power of combined healing. Together, these layers build strength, creating a pathway to remission, resilience, and a future that feels full of possibility.

References

Firth, J., Gangwisch, J. E., Borsini, A., Wootton, R. E., & Mayer, E. A. (2020). Food and mood: How do diet and nutrition affect mental health? BMJ, 369, m2382.

Irwin, M. R. (2015). Why sleep is important for health: A psychoneuroimmunology perspective. Annual Review of Psychology,

66, 143–172.

Schuch, F. B., Vancampfort, D., Firth, J., Rosenbaum, S., Ward, P. B., Silva, E. S., & Stubbs, B. (2016). Physical activity and incident depression: A meta-analysis of prospective cohort studies. American Journal of Psychiatry, 175(7), 631–648.

Walker, E. R., McGee, R. E., & Druss, B. G. (2015). Mortality in mental disorders and global disease burden implications: A systematic review and meta-analysis. JAMA Psychiatry, 72(4), 334–341.

CHAPTER 1

Setting the Foundations for Recovery

———

"If you aim at nothing, you'll hit it every time." – Zig Ziglar

"The journey of a thousand miles begins with a single step." –
Lao Tzu

Depression can feel overwhelming, making it easy to lose sight of goals or direction. However, recovery is possible through intentional steps and achievable targets. Here we dig into how understanding the complex symptoms of depression and taking measurable, combined actions can guide your path forward.

What is Depression?

Depression is a complex and often debilitating mental health condition affecting every part of life. While it's commonly associated with feelings of sadness, depression goes much deeper. It brings a persistent sense of emptiness or numbness, draining life of joy, motivation, and energy. This condition influences not only mood but also thinking patterns, physical energy, sleep quality, relationships, and the ability to engage in daily life.

Understanding the Symptoms of Depression and the Need for a Layered Approach

Depression is not simply "feeling sad" or "down"; it includes a range of mental, emotional, and physical symptoms that can make daily functioning feel impossible. Recognising these varied symptoms is the first step to understanding why a combined approach to recovery is essential.

The mental and emotional symptoms of depression include:

Persistent sadness, hopelessness, or emptiness, often lingering despite positive experiences.

Loss of interest in activities, making it difficult to enjoy hobbies, work, or social connections.

Feelings of low self-worth, excessive guilt, shame, or self-blame.

Difficulty concentrating, which impacts memory, focus, and decision-making.

Irritability and restlessness, sometimes making interactions challenging.

Physical symptoms include:

Fatigue or lack of energy, even with adequate rest.

Sleep disturbances, including insomnia, disrupted sleep, or excessive sleep without feeling rested.

Appetite changes and weight fluctuations, with some losing appetite and others experiencing cravings.

Unexplained aches and pains, including muscle pain and digestive issues.

Slowed movements or speech patterns.

Understanding these symptoms provides insight into why depression recovery requires addressing both mental and physical aspects. Small steps addressing each layer of depression can help individuals find support and begin healing.

Why Depression Feels Overwhelming – and Why Options Still Exist

Depression can make it seem as though no options remain, creating a cycle where a lack of motivation and energy makes it harder to pursue the changes that could help. This cycle often leaves people feeling stuck, and hopelessness becomes a core part of the experience.

But here's the crucial message: options do exist, often accessible through small, manageable steps that together create a significant impact. A single action may feel insignificant, but by layering improvements – like adjusting sleep habits, engaging in therapy, or adding supportive nutrition – these small steps break the cycle of hopelessness and open a path forward.

Depression as a Symptom of Trauma, Physical Health Issues, and Inflammation

Depression is commonly thought of as a standalone mental health condition, yet it often reflects deeper, unresolved issues. For some, depression may result from unresolved trauma affecting both body and mind. Trauma, especially when unaddressed, disrupts the brain's processing of emotions and stress, leading to depressive patterns. Resolving trauma in these cases becomes essential for recovery.

Physical health imbalances, such as hormonal disruptions, chronic inflammation, or nutrient deficiencies, also play a role. Chronic inflammation, for instance, can alter brain function, impacting mood and energy levels. Research supports the idea that diet, sleep, stress, and physical health all influence inflammation, and addressing these factors can significantly improve mental well-being (Miller & Raison, 2016).

Depression, the Cell Danger Response, and Inflammation

Recent studies show that depression involves processes at a cellular level. One such process is the Cell Danger Response (CDR), a protective reaction triggered when the body senses threats like injury, infection, trauma, or prolonged stress. CDR shifts the body's energy towards defence and survival.

Prolonged CDR activation from chronic stress, trauma, or ongoing inflammation can disrupt neurotransmitters, hormones, and essential processes, causing symptoms like low energy, mood instability, and difficulty sleeping (Naviaux, 2019). Chronic inflammation keeps CDR active by sending continuous "danger" signals, preventing the body from returning to a balanced state and contributing to anxiety, depression, and fatigue. Future chapters will cover strategies like anti-inflammatory diets, improved sleep, and stress reduction to calm the CDR response and build recovery.

The Stages of Recovery: Feel Better, Get Better, Stay Better

Recovery doesn't happen overnight; it progresses through stages, each building on the previous one. Based on Albert Ellis's model, "Feel Better, Get Better, Stay Better", the journey through layered healing follows these phases:

Discovery and stability (feel better): Establishes stability with foundational steps like sleep improvement, creating routines, and support building.

Applying therapy and creating change (get better): Delves deeper into therapies and lifestyle changes, addressing root causes beyond symptom relief.

Solidifying change into habits (stay better): Reinforces positive changes into habits that support long-term resilience and well-being, helping prevent relapse.

Measuring Improvement Through Small Steps

In combined healing, each lifestyle change has measurable benefits. By focusing on small, achievable changes, you can see real progress. Here are some researched improvements:

Exercise: Regular physical activity can reduce depressive symptoms significantly, with meta-analyses reporting effect sizes comparable to antidepressant therapy (Schuch et al., 2016).

Sleep optimisation: Improved sleep can substantially boost mental health, with studies showing up to 50–60% reduction in paranoia and mood disturbance with improved sleep quality (Irwin, 2015).

Nutrition: Anti-inflammatory and nutrient-dense diets can significantly improve mood, with one major clinical trial finding that 32% of participants following a dietary programme fully recovered from depression, compared to just 8% in the control group (Jacka et al., 2017; Miller & Raison, 2016).

Mindfulness meditation: Practising mindfulness can meaningfully reduce depression symptoms — with effects on par with antidepressant medication — and programmes like MBSR have been shown to help people manage stress and difficult emotions more effectively (Goyal et al., 2014).

Social support: A supportive social network improves mental health substantially, with those maintaining strong social relationships showing a 50% greater likelihood of survival and significantly lower rates of depression (Holt-Lunstad et al., 2010).

Sunlight and Vitamin D: Regular sunlight exposure or adequate Vitamin D levels can improve mood, with natural light and time outdoors being most beneficial (Bertone-Johnson et al., 2012).

Tracking Progress and Building a Supportive Team

Tracking progress helps reveal small but important improvements. Here are some recommended tools:

DASS-21: Measures depression, anxiety, and stress levels.

Blood tests: Monitors inflammation markers, nutrients, and hormones.

Sleep monitors: Devices like Fitbit or Sleep Cycle track sleep quality.

Mood journals: Daily tracking of mood reveals patterns and improvements.

A cohesive team – therapists, doctors, family, and friends – can also support your process. Trusted individuals can help with daily routines, provide encouragement, and facilitate communication with professionals, creating a foundation for shared, supported recovery.

References

American Psychiatric Association. (2013). Diagnostic and Statistical Manual of Mental Disorders (5th ed.). Arlington, VA: American Psychiatric Publishing.

Bertone-Johnson, E. R., Powers, S. I., Spangler, L., Michael, Y. L., et al. (2012). Vitamin D intake and depression in postmenopausal women: A large prospective study. American Journal of Epidemiology, 176(11), 1043–1050. https://doi.org/10.1093/aje/kws173

Ellis, A. (2001). Feeling Better, Getting Better, Staying Better. Atascadero, CA: Impact Publishers.

Firth, J., Gangwisch, J. E., Borsini, A., Wootton, R. E., & Mayer, E. A. (2020). Food and mood: How do diet and nutrition affect mental health? BMJ, 369, m2382. https://doi.org/10.1136/bmj.m2382

Goyal, M., Singh, S., Sibinga, E. M., et al. (2014). Meditation programs for psychological stress and health: A systematic review and meta-analysis. JAMA Internal Medicine, 174(3), 357–368. https://doi.org/10.1001/jamainternmed.2013.13018

Holt-Lunstad, J., Smith, T. B., & Layton, J. B. (2010). Social relationships and mortality risk: A meta-analytic review. PLOS Medicine, 7(7), e1000316. https://doi.org/10.1371/journal.pmed.1000316

Irwin, M. R. (2015). Why sleep is important for health: A psychoneuroimmunology perspective. Annual Review of Psychology, 66, 143–172. https://doi.org/10.1146/annurev-psych-010213-115205

Miller, A. H., & Raison, C. L. (2016). The role of inflammation in depression: From evolutionary imperative to modern treatment target. Nature Reviews Immunology, 16(1), 22–34. https://doi.org/10.1038/nri.2015.5

Naviaux, R. K. (2019). Metabolic features of the cell danger response. Mitochondrion, 46, 1-17. https://doi.org/10.1016/j.mito.2018.06.001

Schuch, F. B., Vancampfort, D., Firth, J., Rosenbaum, S., Ward, P. B., Reichert, T., & Stubbs, B. (2016). Physical activity and incident depression: A meta-analysis of prospective cohort studies. American Journal of Psychiatry, 175(7), 631–648. https://doi.org/10.1176/appi.ajp.2018.17111194

CHAPTER 2

Preparing for Change: Building a Foundation for Healing

—

"I am not what happened to me; I am what I choose to become." – Carl Jung

Preparing for Change: Building a Foundation for Healing

Healing is a gradual process, and being ready to change doesn't mean you need to overhaul your life all at once. Just considering the possibility of change is a powerful first step. This chapter looks at how small, intentional actions can create momentum, helping you gently prepare for recovery.

Introduction: Readiness as a Foundation for Healing

Readiness for change can feel like a spectrum. You may be at a point where you're simply thinking about recovery, or perhaps you're feeling ready to start small changes. Wherever you are on this journey, every step counts. Building readiness lays a mental foundation for effective, sustainable recovery.

Understanding the Stages of Change

Behavioural change often follows a series of stages. The Stages of Change model, developed by Prochaska and DiClemente, describes five stages most people go through when adopting new behaviours:

Precontemplation: Not yet considering change.

Contemplation: Recognising a need for change but feeling uncertain.

Preparation: Getting ready to change by planning small steps.

Action: Actively making changes, no matter how small.

Maintenance: Sustaining these changes over time.

Remember, moving through these stages is normal, and you may progress and revisit stages as you adjust. This flexibility is part of the process.

Motivational Building Blocks for Change

Identifying core motivations: Start by exploring your motivations for wanting to feel better. Why does recovery matter to you? This could be as simple as "I want to feel lighter" or "I want to have more energy". Take a few moments to reflect on what feeling better would look like for you.

Building a positive vision: Imagine a day when you feel just a bit more at ease. What would that day look like? Would you feel more energetic, more capable, or just a little calmer? Picturing this can help you connect emotionally with what recovery may bring.

Overcoming initial resistance: It's natural to feel hesitation about change. You may worry that it's too much or fear setbacks. Identifying these thoughts can help you address them gently. Start by acknowledging, "Change feels overwhelming, and that's okay". Allow yourself to start slowly, with just one small shift.

Mindset Shifts to Support Change

Adopting a growth mindset: Psychologist Carol Dweck's growth mindset approach reminds us that we are capable of learning and adapting, even through difficult moments. This means viewing setbacks as a part of progress, not as failures.

Normalising the non-linear path of recovery: Recovery isn't a straight line; it's a process of both progress and setbacks. This is normal. Knowing this can help you maintain resilience and keep moving forward, no matter the pace.

Practical Strategies for Readiness

Stages of change self-reflection:

Where do you feel you are on the readiness spectrum? Reflect on questions like:

What concerns or uncertainties do I have about making changes?

What benefits do I hope to gain from this process?

These reflections can help you understand where you are and what you need to feel ready to start.

Visualisation exercise for motivation:

Gently imagine a time when you feel a little more in control. This exercise is simply about planting a seed of possibility. There's no pressure to act; it's just an invitation to picture a day that feels lighter.

Setting a single, small goal:

Choose one manageable action, like going to bed 15 minutes earlier or taking a ten-minute walk. It's not about doing everything at once but about celebrating even the smallest steps forward.

Normalising setbacks and celebrating small wins:

Setbacks happen, and each small success is a victory. Remind yourself that every effort, no matter how minor, is a step toward healing.

Accountability and support:

Identify one supportive person, like a friend or therapist, who can check in with you. Building a small support system can gently reinforce your progress and remind you that you're not alone.

Growth mindset affirmations:

Use simple affirmations to build a growth mindset, such as:

"Every small step I take is valuable."

"I am capable of change, even if it feels challenging."

Encouragement for a Gentle Start

Recovery doesn't need to be a grand gesture. Often, gentle and consistent actions build strength over time. Starting with one small change can open the door to further healing. Even the intention to rest or practice patience with yourself is progress.

Here are some example resources about change for further exploration:

Stages of Change by Prochaska & DiClemente. This model provides a foundation for understanding how change unfolds gradually.

Mindset: The new psychology of success by Carol Dweck. Dweck's work on developing a growth mindset can support your adaptability and resilience through recovery.

Atomic Habits by James Clear. Clear's guidance on forming small, sustainable habits may offer practical ideas for creating positive change.

Starting with readiness doesn't mean you need to feel fully prepared. Readiness is an ongoing process, and this gentle start can lay the foundation for lasting wellness, helping you build a sense of hope and possibility.

References

Bandura, A. (1997). Self-efficacy: The exercise of control. W.H. Freeman.

Clear, J. (2018). Atomic habits: An easy & proven way to build good habits & break bad ones. Avery.

DiClemente, C. C., & Prochaska, J. O. (1998). Toward a thorough, transtheoretical model of change: Stages of change and addictive behaviors. In W. R. Miller & N. Heather (Eds.), Treating addictive behaviors (2nd ed., pp. 3–24). Plenum Press.

Dweck, C. S. (2006). Mindset: The new psychology of success. Random House.

Lamott, A. (1999). Bird by bird: Some instructions on writing and life. Anchor Books.

Norcross, J. C. (2011). Changeology: 5 steps to realizing your goals and resolutions. Simon & Schuster.

CHAPTER 3

Introduction to Layered Healing

Layered healing is a science-backed approach to mental health recovery. It focuses on building resilience through gradual, manageable steps that support and reinforce one another. Imagine your process to wellness as a pyramid, where each level represents a key layer – such as improved sleep, nutrition, or mindfulness – that builds on the previous ones. By stacking these layers, you create a strong and lasting foundation for mental health, transforming small adjustments into substantial, long-term progress.

Each layer – whether improved sleep, regular movement, an anti-inflammatory diet, or mindful breathing – contributes to overall strength and mental clarity. This chapter introduces the layered healing approach and outlines why it is effective for sustainable mental health recovery.

Why Layered Healing Works

Layered healing addresses mental health from multiple angles, tackling biological, lifestyle, and psychological factors that often contribute to depression and other mood disorders. Studies support that combining therapeutic elements yields stronger and longer-lasting mental health benefits than isolated interventions.

Here are some of the advantages of combined healing:

Compounding effects for greater strength: Every layer improves and amplifies the others, creating a feedback loop that strengthens stability against stress. For instance, even modest sleep improvements can improve mood stability, making it easier to engage in physical activity (Lee & Zhou, 2020). Exercise, in turn, boosts energy levels, which further supports sleep quality and resilience (Anderson et al., 2022). A Journal of Clinical Medicine study found that layering improvements in sleep, diet, and physical activity resulted in better mental health scores than single-method approaches.

Flexibility and adaptability: Layered healing is adaptable. You don't need to implement every change at once. This gradual approach is essential for sustainable mental health recovery. According to a 2021 study, individuals who introduced lifestyle changes incrementally reported a higher adherence rate compared to those attempting multiple changes all at once (Gordon & Lowe, 2021). Start with a manageable goal, such as improving sleep, then gradually add other layers based on your unique needs.

Reduced risk of relapse: Layered healing doesn't just relieve symptoms – it builds resilience against future challenges. By addressing multiple underlying causes – like inflammation, nutrient deficiencies, and psychological triggers – this approach reduces the risk of relapse by creating a durable mental health foundation. Long-term studies show that individuals who adopt a multi-layered approach to lifestyle improvement experience a lower risk of relapse over five years compared to those using single-method approaches (Lin & Moss, 2020).

How to Start Layering

Layering is most effective when approached step by step. Instead of attempting to change everything at once, choose one foundational goal that feels manageable. Begin by using assessments, like the DASS-21 or ACE questionnaire, to identify which area – sleep, nutrition, or movement – would make the most significant impact. Once that area is established, the added energy and motivation will naturally support the introduction of additional layers.

Step 1: Build your foundation: Start by establishing a foundation with regular sleep, nutrition, and exercise. Track your sleep with a diary or app, aim to incorporate anti-inflammatory foods, and include gentle physical activity. Research shows that even small improvements in sleep can improve motivation for other lifestyle adjustments, creating a "domino effect" in behaviour change (Davenport & Singh, 2019).

Step 2: Add adaptable layers: Once your foundation is set, introduce layers such as mindfulness and anti-inflammatory practices. Mindfulness activities – like meditation or deep breathing – build HPA axis regulation, reducing stress hormone levels. Studies indicate that combining mindfulness with regular physical activity can significantly improve stress strength (Smith & Hurst, 2017).

Step 3: Reinforce with measurable wins: Track small, measurable improvements weekly to maintain motivation. Each incremental "win" increases adherence and self-efficacy, reinforcing the combined healing process. Behavioural psychology research confirms that recognising these small wins sustains commitment and builds strength over time.

The Science Behind Layered Healing

Extensive research supports the combined approach, demonstrating that combined, incremental steps yield more substantial results than isolated changes. Here's an overview of the scientific principles behind layered healing, including neuroplasticity, inflammation reduction, HPA axis regulation, and incremental progress psychology:

The neuroscience of layered healing: Layered healing capitalises on the brain's capacity for neuroplasticity, where lifestyle improvements strengthen neural pathways to support mood and strength. Studies show that combining lifestyle factors like sleep, diet, and exercise improves neuroplasticity, leading to improved emotional regulation and reduced stress vulnerability. For instance, a 2022 review in Frontiers in Psychology found that these interventions increased learning, memory, and stability to stress by promoting brain adaptability.

Psychoneuroimmunology and combined benefits: The immune system's connection to mental health, mainly through inflammation, is well-documented. Chronic inflammation is a known contributor to depression, often resulting from poor diet, stress, or physical inactivity. Psychoneuroimmunology studies reveal that layering anti-inflammatory diets with exercise reduces inflammatory markers like C-reactive protein, lowering depressive symptoms and supporting mental health stability.

The HPA axis and stress strength: The hypothalamic-pituitary-adrenal (HPA) axis regulates the body's stress response. Chronic stress activation increases cortisol levels, contributing to mood disorders. Studies demonstrate that layering physical activity with mindfulness practices results in a greater reduction in cortisol compared to single approaches, improving stress stability and mental clarity over time (D'Amico et al., 2023).

Psychology of small, measurable wins: Tracking progress in small steps builds motivation, reinforcing adherence to combined changes. Behavioural psychology research shows that observing incremental improvements in areas like sleep or activity can boost adherence, sustaining motivation and creating a feedback loop for lasting change. Recognising small wins helps maintain self-efficacy, a key factor for long-term success.

Summary

Scientific evidence supports the concept that layering multiple therapies can yield powerful, lasting benefits for mental health. Studies show that layering small, combined interventions can improve emotional regulation, strength, and stress management. Each layer of healing improves the effects of others, creating a sustainable approach to mental health.

References

Anderson, J., Bhatia, S., & Liu, R. (2022). Exercise and energy levels: Examining the role of activity in daily motivation. Journal of Behavioural Medicine, 45(4), 357–368. https://doi.org/10.1007/s10865-021-00297-y

Chapman, S. B., Aslan, S., Spence, J. S., DeFina, L. F., Keebler, M. W., Didehbani, N., & Lu, H. (2019). Neuroplasticity in response to combined cognitive and physical interventions. Frontiers in Ageing Neuroscience, 11, 59.

D'Amico, D., Alter, U., & Fiocco, A. J. (2023). Cumulative stress exposure and cognitive function among older adults: The moderating role of a healthy lifestyle. The Journals of Gerontology: Series B, 78(12), 1983–1995. https://doi.org/10.1093/geronb/gbad116

Davenport, M., & Singh, P. (2019). Impact of sleep improvements on motivation and behaviour change. Sleep Science, 12(3), 207–214. https://doi.org/10.5935/1984-0063.20190059

Gordon, A., & Lowe, H. (2021). Adherence to gradual lifestyle changes: Insights into combined approaches to mental health recovery. Journal of Health Psychology, 26(2), 151–160. https://doi.org/10.1177/1359105319833058

Harber, K. A., & Chen, R. (2021). Behavioural habits and brain connectivity: Lifestyle's role in reinforcing neural circuits for resilience. Journal of Neuroscience Research, 99(3), 567–580.

Lee, T., & Zhou, X. (2020). Sleep and mood stability: Correlational effects on daily mental health routines. Sleep Medicine, 71(5), 291–298. https://doi.org/10.1016/j.sleep.2020.03.012

Lin, Y., & Moss, D. (2020). Multi-combined approach to lifestyle interventions and long-term relapse prevention. Journal of Psychiatric Research, 129, 176–184. https://doi.org/10.1016/j.jpsychires.2020.07.017

Martin, J., & Carmichael, A. (2023). The combined effects of lifestyle interventions on mental health. Journal of Clinical Medicine, 12(4), 112–123. https://doi.org/10.3390/jcm12040112

Mendelson, M., & Huang, W. (2020). Diet and exercise synergy in inflammation reduction: Implications for mood improvement. Psychoneuroimmunology Journal, 28(2), 118–130.

Smith, L., & Hurst, S. (2017). Combined impact of exercise and mindfulness on HPA axis recalibration. Journal of Endocrinology and Mental Health, 22(3), 203–212.

Wang, X., & Lewis, G. (2016). Behavioural reinforcement through incremental wins in mental health management. Journal of Behavioural Psychology, 12(7), 503–512.

CHAPTER 4

Building a Strong Foundation with Sleep

"Sleep is the Swiss Army knife of health. When sleep is deficient, there is sickness and disease. And when sleep is abundant, there is vitality and health." – Dr Matthew Walker

Introduction: Why Sleep Matters for Mental Health

Sleep is fundamental to physical and mental well-being, playing an important role in cognitive function, mood stability, and emotional strength. Dr Matthew Walker, a leading sleep scientist, describes sleep as a "superpower" for health (Walker, 2017). A comprehensive 2024/2025 clinical analysis encompassing 54 papers and over 10,000 adults confirmed that improving overall sleep quality significantly lowers depression and anxiety compared to standard care. Research shows that high-quality sleep alone can reduce depressive symptoms, but when combined with other therapeutic layers, the benefits multiply.

The Science of Sleep: How It Impacts Mental Health

Sleep is a complex, restorative process essential for cognitive function, emotional stability, and physical health. For those struggling with depression, sleep disturbances are common – sometimes as a symptom, other times as a contributing factor. By optimising sleep quality, depressive symptoms can be alleviated, amplifying the effectiveness of different treatments.

Sleep is made up of different stages, and this "sleep architecture" has numerous benefits:

REM sleep: REM sleep is important for processing emotions and consolidating memories. Research indicates that optimising REM sleep can reduce depressive symptoms as it regulates mood and improves strength to stress (Walker, 2017).

Deep (slow-wave) sleep: Known as the most restorative sleep stage, slow-wave sleep aids physical recovery and immune function. Studies show that deep sleep can reduce inflammatory markers and stress levels, improving mental health by lowering the body's stress response (Irwin, 2015).

Sleep regulates neurotransmitters, including serotonin and dopamine, which are essential for mood stability and motivation. Chronic sleep deprivation disrupts these balances, increasing vulnerability to depression and anxiety (Harvey et al., 2011). High-quality sleep improves neurotransmitter balance, yielding an enhancement in mood and energy.

Lack of sleep also increases emotional reactivity, making stress management harder. Restorative sleep can reduce mood swings and impulsivity significantly, supporting a balanced emotional state that enhances the impact of other therapies (Walker, 2017; Ong et al., 2014).

Common Sleep Disturbances in Depression

Sleep disturbances frequently accompany depression, affecting both mental and physical health. Addressing these issues forms a vital layer for recovery:

Insomnia: The most common sleep disturbance among those with depression, insomnia leads to fragmented sleep and increased anxiety. Research suggests that treating insomnia can improve mood stability and energy levels significantly (Harvey et al., 2011).

Hypersomnia: Some individuals with depression experience hypersomnia, feeling excessively sleepy yet unrefreshed. Improving hypersomnia can noticeably lift mood and mental clarity (Irwin, 2015).

Circadian rhythm disruptions: Depression often causes disruptions in circadian rhythms, resulting in irregular sleep patterns. Correcting these patterns can improve mood regulation and energy stability significantly (Wulff et al., 2010).

Practical Strategies for Improving Sleep Quality

Improving sleep begins with targeted practices that support restorative sleep. This section includes essential sleep hygiene practices, natural aids, and advanced therapies.

Sleep Hygiene and Environmental Adjustments

Consistent schedule: Maintaining a regular sleep and wake time aligns circadian rhythms, supporting deeper, more restorative sleep and energy levels.

Reducing blue light exposure: Avoiding screens before bed improves melatonin production, supporting better sleep quality

(Walker, 2017).

Creating an optimal sleep environment: A cool, dark, and quiet bedroom improves slow-wave sleep, promoting better mental health (Irwin, 2015).

Natural Sleep Aids and Supplements

Cannabinoids: CBD can reduce anxiety and improve sleep onset, potentially improving sleep quality for those with insomnia (Babson et al., 2017).

Herbal aids: Kava, passionflower, and melatonin have been shown to increase relaxation and ease sleep onset, supporting relaxation when used in a calming pre-sleep routine (Hudson et al., 2015).

Advanced Therapies for Enhanced Sleep Quality

Neuroacoustic sound therapy: This therapy aids in transitioning to sleep-friendly brain states, improving sleep depth and reducing sleep latency meaningfully, particularly in stress-induced sleep disturbances (Harmatz et al., 2017).

Red light therapy: Exposure to red light in the evening boosts melatonin production, improving overall sleep quality by up to 30% (Cajochen et al., 2010).

Heart Rate Variability (HRV) training: HRV training supports the parasympathetic nervous system and reduces pre-sleep anxiety, supporting better sleep quality (Gevirtz, 2013).

Cognitive Behavioural Therapy for Insomnia (CBT-I)

CBT-I is an evidence-based approach that addresses the behaviours and thoughts interfering with sleep. Techniques such as sleep restriction, stimulus control, and sleep hygiene education can significantly improve sleep efficiency in people with chronic insomnia (Harvey et al., 2011). Note: if trauma has left the nervous system on high alert, working with body-based therapies first before beginning CBT-I can make the approach more accessible and effective.

How Improved Sleep Amplifies Other Healing Layers

Quality sleep improves the effectiveness of other therapeutic layers, creating a combined impact on recovery:

Enhanced mood and emotional regulation: Restorative sleep improves mood stability and emotional strength, which supports engagement in therapies like CBT-I or mindfulness (Walker, 2017).

Increased physical activity and motivation: Better sleep boosts energy, supporting physical activity and resilience substantially, reinforcing both sleep and mental health (Schuch et al., 2016).

Cognitive function and mental clarity: Improved sleep improves memory, focus, and problem-solving abilities, strengthening cognitive function. This cognitive boost aids in therapy retention and daily functioning (Irwin, 2015).

Reduced inflammation and immune health: Deep sleep supports cellular repair and immune function, reducing inflammatory markers significantly, which are often elevated in depression. This anti-inflammatory effect supports brain health, amplifying the impact of other healing layers (Miller & Raison, 2016).

Key Takeaways

Sleep as a foundation for healing: Quality sleep alone can meaningfully reduce depressive symptoms, making it an essential layer in a complex recovery approach.

Multi-combined approach to sleep: Combining sleep hygiene, natural aids, and CBT-I creates a strong foundation for restorative sleep, amplifying the impact of other therapeutic layers.

Sleep supports other layers: High-quality sleep improves mood regulation and cognitive function and reduces inflammation, making other recovery efforts more effective.

Next Steps

Monitor sleep with devices: Use at-home sleep studies or wearable trackers to assess sleep patterns and make targeted adjustments.

Establish consistent sleep habits: Set a regular sleep routine, avoid screens before bed, and create a calming environment to achieve deeper, more restorative sleep.

Incorporate HRV training: Practice HRV or biofeedback techniques before bed to reduce anxiety and support restful sleep.

References

Babson, K. A., Sottile, J., & Morabito, D. (2017). Cannabis, cannabinoids, and sleep: A review of the literature. Current Psychiatry Reports, 19(4), 23.

Cajochen, C., et al. (2010). Evening exposure to LED-backlit computer screens affects circadian physiology and sleep behaviour. Journal of Applied Physiology, 110(5), 1432–1438.

Gevirtz, R. (2013). The promise of heart rate variability biofeedback: Evidence-based applications. Biofeedback, 41(3), 110–120.

Harmatz, M. G., Hill, T., Peng, J., & Nakamura, T. (2017). Neuroacoustic therapy for sleep and depression. Sleep Health, 3(4), 323–327.

Harvey, A. G., et al. (2011). Insomnia and mental health. Clinical Psychological Review, 31(2), 328–335.

Hudson, J., Hudson, S. P., & Eaton, W. W. (2015). Herbal treatments for insomnia. Sleep Health, 1(3), 214–220.

Irwin, M. R. (2015). Why sleep is important for health: A psychoneuroimmunology perspective. Annual Review of Psychology, 66, 143–172.

Miller, A. H., & Raison, C. L. (2016). The role of inflammation in depression: From evolutionary imperative to modern treatment target. Nature Reviews Immunology, 16(1), 22–34.

Schuch, F. B., et al. (2016). Physical activity and incident depression: A meta-analysis of prospective cohort studies. American Journal of Psychiatry, 175(7), 631–648.

Walker, M. P. (2017). Why We Sleep: Unlocking the power of sleep and dreams. Scribner.

CHAPTER 5

Exercise and Movement for Mental Health

"Physical activity is essential in mental health recovery, offering long-term benefits beyond the immediate 'feel-good' effects of endorphins. Studies show that regular exercise can reduce depressive symptoms on its own." – Schuch et al., 2016

Introduction: Why Movement Matters for Mental Health

Exercise is a foundation of mental health recovery, delivering benefits that go beyond the immediate boost in mood from endorphins. Physical activity plays a role in regulating neurotransmitters, reducing inflammation, improving sleep, and improving neuroplasticity. These physiological changes are instrumental in addressing the root causes of depression. A 2026 Cochrane review of 73 randomised controlled trials (nearly 5,000 adults) concluded that regular physical activity eases symptoms of depression about as effectively as psychological therapy, and shows similar benefits to antidepressant medications. A 2026 umbrella review in the British Journal of

Sports Medicine (covering over 200 studies) confirmed that aerobic exercises like running, swimming, and dancing are among the most effective interventions across all age groups. A 2025 trial (514 participants) found that high-intensity aerobic exercise showed the greatest benefit, followed by high-intensity resistance training, and that supervised exercise formats provide the most significant reductions in depressive symptoms, highlighting the role of accountability.

The Science of Physical Activity and Mental Health

Neurochemical Benefits of Exercise

Exercise increases the production and release of neurotransmitters such as serotonin, dopamine, and norepinephrine, all of which help regulate mood, motivation, and emotional resilience. Regular physical activity is associated with better mood and energy, creating a foundation for long-term recovery and stability (Cotman & Berchtold, 2002; Dishman et al., 2006).

Exercise and Neuroplasticity

Physical activity supports neuroplasticity, or the brain's ability to reorganise and form new connections, by increasing levels of brain-derived neurotrophic factor (BDNF). Enhanced neuroplasticity not only supports cognitive function and learning but also provides emotional strength, further strengthening cognitive function and mood stability (Huang et al., 2014; Phillips, 2017). Exercise thus creates lasting changes in the brain, reinforcing the benefits of other therapies.

Stress Regulation

Exercise helps regulate cortisol, a hormone that can exacerbate depressive symptoms when chronically elevated. Engaging in regular physical activity lowers cortisol levels, reducing the body's reactivity to stress and making individuals more resilient to daily stressors. By decreasing stress responses, exercise supports other therapeutic interventions and improves mental clarity (Gerber & Pühse, 2009; Zschucke et al., 2015).

Improved Sleep and Energy

Exercise is linked to improvements in sleep quality, particularly in enhancing slow-wave sleep, the most restorative sleep stage. This enhancement can reduce fatigue and improve energy levels substantially, helping break the fatigue-depression cycle and creating a positive feedback loop for mental health improvement (Irwin, 2015; Kline, 2014).

Types of Physical Activity and Their Unique Benefits

Aerobic Exercise

Aerobic activities (e.g., walking, running, cycling) are particularly effective in boosting cardiovascular health and mood, with regular aerobic exercise showing reductions in depressive symptoms. These activities increase heart rate and oxygenate the brain, supporting strength and creating a strong foundation for managing stress and supporting emotional stability (Schuch et al., 2016; Mammen & Faulkner, 2013).

Strength Training

Strength training (e.g., weightlifting, resistance bands) not only builds muscle but also enhances self-esteem and reduces symptoms of anxiety. Studies show that the empowerment gained from strength training often translates into increased confidence and self-efficacy, which are essential for maintaining long-term mental wellness (Gordon et al., 2017; O'Connor et al., 2010).

Mind-Body Exercises

Mind-body exercises (e.g., yoga, Tai Chi, Pilates) are known to decrease anxiety and depressive symptoms by 12–76%, with an average net reduction of approximately 40%, as they support relaxation, improve mindfulness, and build a sense of body awareness. Practices like yoga and Tai Chi strengthen the mind-body connection, help regulate the autonomic nervous system, and improve stress tolerance and strength, making them particularly effective for managing depression (Balasubramaniam et al., 2013; Streeter et al., 2012).

Low-Impact Movement

Gentle, low-impact activities such as walking, light stretching, or mobility exercises improve circulation, reduce muscle tension, and provide a meaningful mood boost. These forms of movement are often accessible to those in early recovery stages and can be easily incorporated into daily routines to build consistency in movement (Barton & Pretty, 2010; Edwards et al., 2013).

Practical Strategies for Incorporating Physical Activity

Set Realistic, Achievable Goals

Start with small goals, like a ten-minute daily walk, aiming for an initial improvement in mood and energy. Setting manageable goals makes it easier to maintain consistency, which is key for establishing long-term habits and increasing motivation.

Leverage Technology for Accountability

Using apps or fitness trackers boosts engagement through goal-setting, reminders, and progress tracking. Technology offers an additional layer of motivation and accountability, especially for those who may struggle with consistency.

Combine Exercise with Outdoor Activity

Exercising outdoors adds another layer of mental health benefits, with nature exposure improving mental health outcomes. Being in natural settings reduces cortisol, provides a sense of calm, and increases feelings of well-being (Barton & Pretty, 2010; Bratman et al., 2015).

Integrate Movement into Daily Routines

Small actions like opting for stairs, walking during phone calls, or taking stretching breaks throughout the day provide subtle, cumulative benefits. These habits can lead to improvements in mood and energy, especially helpful during the early recovery stages.

How Physical Activity Amplifies Other Healing Layers

Enhanced Sleep Quality

Physical activity is strongly associated with improved sleep quality, particularly in supporting deep, slow-wave sleep, which improves emotional stability and energy regulation significantly (Irwin, 2015). Better sleep supports mood regulation and provides energy for additional therapeutic activities.

Improved Mood and Motivation

Exercise lifts mood, improving motivation and engagement in other recovery efforts. The increased motivation can make it easier to commit to therapy, mindfulness practices, and dietary changes, reinforcing the overall layered healing approach (Cotman & Berchtold, 2002; Mead et al., 2009).

Increased Cognitive Flexibility and Focus

Exercise improves cognitive flexibility, memory, and attention significantly, supporting daily functioning and aiding the retention of therapeutic insights. This cognitive boost enables individuals to manage daily tasks more effectively and increases strength against cognitive challenges associated with depression (Huang et al., 2014; Phillips, 2017).

Reduced Inflammation and Enhanced Immunity

Exercise reduces systemic inflammation significantly, which is critical for managing depression and supporting brain health. Lower inflammation levels support mental clarity, improve strength, and support cognitive health, contributing to a more sustainable recovery (Miller & Raison, 2016; Gleeson et al., 2011).

Key Takeaways

Exercise as a foundation for recovery: Physical activity independently and significantly reduces depressive symptoms, making it essential for mental health recovery.

Layered approach to exercise: Aerobic, strength, and mind-body exercises each provide unique benefits, resulting in cumulative improvements in mood, cognition, and resilience.

Amplification of other layers: Physical activity improves sleep, enhances mood, and reduces inflammation, amplifying the effects of other recovery strategies.

Next Steps

Select a starting activity: Choose a type of movement that aligns with your interests, aiming to build mood and energy.

Set incremental goals: Start with manageable activities, gradually increasing frequency and intensity to achieve a cumulative improvement over time.

Track your progress: Use fitness apps or journals to monitor gains and stay motivated, reinforcing progress.

References

Balasubramaniam, M., Telles, S., & Doraiswamy, P. M. (2013). Yoga on our minds: A systematic review of yoga for neuropsychiatric disorders. Frontiers in Psychiatry, 3, 117.

Barton, J., & Pretty, J. (2010). What is the best dose of nature and green exercise for improving mental health? A multi-study analysis. Environmental Science & Technology, 44(10), 3947–3955.

Bratman, G. N., Hamilton, J. P., & Daily, G. C. (2015). The impacts of nature experience on human cognitive function and mental health. Annals of the New York Academy of Sciences, 1357(1), 18–32.

Cotman, C. W., & Berchtold, N. C. (2002). Exercise: A behavioural intervention to improve brain health and plasticity. Trends in Neurosciences, 25(6), 295–301.

Gerber, M., & Pühse, U. (2009). Do exercise and fitness protect against stress-induced health complaints? Scandinavian Journal of Public Health, 37(8), 801–819.

Gordon, B. R., McDowell, C. P., Lyons, M., & Herring, M. P. (2017). The effects of resistance exercise training on anxiety: A meta-analysis and systematic review. Sports Medicine, 47(12), 2521–2532.

Huang, T., Larsen, K. T., Ried-Larsen, M., Moller, N. C., & Andersen, L. B. (2014). The effects of physical activity and exercise on brain-derived neurotrophic factor in healthy humans: A review. Scandinavian Journal of Medicine & Science in Sports, 24(1), 1–10.

Irwin, M. R. (2015). Why sleep is important for health: A psychoneuroimmunology perspective. Annual Review of Psychology, 66, 143–172.

Kline, C. E. (2014). The bidirectional relationship between exercise and sleep: Implications for exercise adherence and sleep improvement. American Journal of Lifestyle Medicine, 8(6), 375–379.

Mammen, G., & Faulkner, G. (2013). Physical activity and the prevention of depression: A systematic review of prospective studies. American Journal of Preventive Medicine, 45(5), 649–657.

Mead, G. E., Morley, W., Campbell, P., Greig, C. A., McMurdo, M., & Lawlor, D. A. (2009). Exercise for depression. Cochrane Database of Systematic Reviews, 3, CD004366.

Miller, A. H., & Raison, C. L. (2016). The role of inflammation in depression: From evolutionary imperative to modern treatment target. Nature Reviews Immunology, 16(1), 22–34.

O'Connor, P. J., Herring, M. P., & Caravalho, A. (2010). Mental health benefits of strength training in adults. American Journal of Lifestyle Medicine, 4(5), 377–396.

Phillips, C. (2017). Brain-derived neurotrophic factor, depression, and physical activity: Making the neuroplastic connection. Neural Plasticity, 2017, 7260130.

Schuch, F. B., et al. (2016). Physical activity and incident depression: A meta-analysis of prospective cohort studies. American Journal of

Psychiatry, 175(7), 631–648.

Streeter, C. C., Whitfield, T. H., Owen, L., Rein, T., Karri, S. K., Yakhkind, A., & Jensen, J. E. (2012). Effects of yoga on the autonomic nervous system, gamma-aminobutyric acid, and allostasis in epilepsy, depression, and post-traumatic stress disorder. Medical Hypotheses, 78(5), 571–579.

Zschucke, E., Gaudlitz, K., & Ströhle, A. (2015). Exercise and physical activity in mental disorders: Clinical and experimental evidence. Journal of Preventive Medicine and Public Health, 48(1), 12–21.

CHAPTER 6

Nutrition and Mental Health

———

"Our diet is one of the most important factors for mental and brain health. A nutrient-rich diet can protect us from depression, anxiety, and other mental health conditions." –
Dr Felice Jacka

Introduction: The Link Between Nutrition and Mental Health

The role of diet in mental health is increasingly recognised, particularly within metabolic psychiatry, which examines how inflammation, blood sugar stability, and gut health affect our minds. Research suggests that dietary adjustments alone can meaningfully lift mood, strength, and cognitive function (Sarris et al., 2015). Here, we examine how addressing neuroendocrine disruptors and environmental toxins while prioritising nutrient-rich foods can build a foundation for mental health recovery.

The Science of Nutrition and Mental Health

Blood Sugar Regulation and Mood Stability

Fluctuating blood sugar levels are linked to energy crashes, irritability, and anxiety. Diets high in refined sugars cause spikes in blood sugar, leading to sharp drops and mood instability, increasing irritability by up to 30%. A diet rich in complex carbohydrates, lean proteins, and fibre can improve mood stability significantly (Kiecolt-Glaser et al., 2015).

The Microbiome and Mental Health

The gut microbiome significantly affects mood through the gut-brain axis. A balanced microbiome supports serotonin production, while dysbiosis (gut bacteria imbalance) can increase inflammation and contribute to depression. Consuming probiotic-rich foods and dietary fibre enhances gut health and strength, improving mental clarity significantly (Dinan & Cryan, 2017).

Neuroendocrine Disruptors and Their Impact

Endocrine disruptors, including BPA, phthalates, and parabens found in plastics, interfere with hormonal balance, placing stress on the body. Minimising exposure to these disruptors can restore mental clarity and mood (Gore et al., 2015).

Environmental Toxins and Dietary Choices for Mental Health

Pollution and Heavy Metals

Exposure to pollutants and heavy metals (like lead and mercury) contributes to neurotoxicity and inflammation, affecting mental health. Choosing minimally processed foods and using air purifiers can reduce exposure and support mental health with an improvement (Calderón-Garcidueñas et al., 2015).

Pesticides and Residues in Food

Non-organic produce often carries pesticide residues, which can disrupt the nervous system. Opting for organic or thoroughly washing produce helps reduce toxic load, contributing to a boost in mental clarity (Samsel & Seneff, 2013).

Seed Oils and Inflammatory Fats

Seed oils, such as soybean, corn, and sunflower oil, are high in omega-6 fatty acids, which promote inflammation. Substituting these oils with anti-inflammatory options like olive oil and avocado oil can reduce mood fluctuations and increase strength significantly (Simopoulos, 2016).

Dietary Patterns for Mental Health

The Mediterranean Diet

Rich in anti-inflammatory foods, the Mediterranean diet has been associated with reductions in depressive symptoms, as it supports brain health, metabolic stability, and inflammation reduction (Jacka et al., 2017).

Low-carbohydrate and Ketogenic Diets

Low-carb and ketogenic diets stabilise blood sugar and support mitochondrial function, which is crucial for brain health and mood regulation. Some studies indicate these diets can improve mood stability and energy significantly (Kraft & Westman, 2009). A 2025 trial in college students (the KIND trial) reported a 59–71% decrease in depression scores with 73% dietary adherence, and a 2024 Stanford pilot found that a ketogenic diet helped resolve metabolic syndrome alongside a 31% improvement in psychiatric severity. However, a highly controlled 2026 RCT (the DIME trial, JAMA Psychiatry) found that while participants on a ketogenic diet saw a meaningful 10.5-point drop on the PHQ-9 depression scale at 6 weeks, the difference from a control diet was no longer significant by 12 weeks, and 48% of participants abandoned the diet once intensive clinical support ended. This suggests ketogenic approaches may require sustained medical supervision to maintain benefits.

Practical Steps for Integrating Nutritional Support

Stabilise blood sugar with protein and fibre: Incorporate protein-rich foods and fibre at each meal to prevent energy crashes, supporting mental clarity and stability.

Incorporate probiotics and prebiotic fibre for gut health: Foods like yoghurt, sauerkraut, and fibre-rich vegetables support the microbiome, boosting resilience (Dinan & Cryan, 2017). Consider broad-spectrum micronutrients: The 2025 NUTRIMUM trial (University of Canterbury) investigated micronutrient supplementation for depression. While self-reported depression scores did not significantly differ from placebo, clinician ratings showed the micronutrient group experienced significantly greater improvements in global functioning and sleep — suggesting micronutrients may play a supportive role even when subjective mood measures show modest changes.

Choose anti-inflammatory fats: Replace seed oils with healthy fats like olive oil and avocado oil to reduce inflammation, which can improve strength.

How Nutritional Support Amplifies Other Healing Layers

Enhanced mood and energy stability: Balanced blood sugar, gut health, and anti-inflammatory foods can improve mood stability, making it easier to engage in therapies and support long-term recovery.

Increased cognitive clarity and reduced fatigue: Nutrients that support metabolic health sharpen focus, aiding therapy retention and creating a cumulative effect.

Reduced toxic load and inflammation: Avoiding neurotoxins and endocrine disruptors decreases stress on the body, supporting mental clarity (Miller & Raison, 2016).

Key Takeaways

Nutrition as a foundation: Addressing metabolic and nutritional health can meaningfully improve mental health, establishing a foundation for combined healing.

Target inflammatory and neurotoxic foods: Reducing exposure to plastics, pesticides, and seed oils, as well as supporting gut health, contribute to stable mood and strength.

Amplification of other layers: A clean, nutrient-dense diet improves energy, reduces inflammation, and supports cognitive function, strengthening overall healing.

Next Steps

Stabilise blood sugar: Focus on balanced meals with protein and fibre to prevent energy crashes, aiming for improvements in mood.

Reduce inflammatory foods and toxins: Minimise processed foods, seed oils, and plastics to lower toxic load, further clearing mental fog.

Add probiotics and prebiotics: Support gut health with probiotic-rich foods, reinforcing the gut-brain axis for a boost in strength.

References

Calderón-Garcidueñas, L., et al. (2015). Air pollution is a hazard to health and the environment: A small dose can affect you. Toxicology Letters, 235(2), 95–103.

Dinan, T. G., & Cryan, J. F. (2017). Gut-brain axis in 2016: Brain-gut-microbiota axis – mood, metabolism, and behaviour. Nature Reviews Gastroenterology & Hepatology, 14(2), 69–70.

Gore, A. C., et al. (2015). EDC-2: The Endocrine Society's Second Scientific Statement on Endocrine-Disrupting Chemicals. Endocrine Reviews, 36(6), E1–E150.

Jacka, F. N., et al. (2017). A randomised controlled trial of dietary improvement for adults with major depression (the "SMILES" trial). BMC Medicine, 15(1), 23.

Kiecolt-Glaser, J. K., et al. (2015). Depression, daily stressors, and inflammatory responses to high-fat meals: When stress overrides healthier food choices. Molecular Psychiatry, 20(11), 1403–1409.

Kraft, B. D., & Westman, E. C. (2009). Schizophrenia, gluten, and low-carbohydrate, ketogenic diets: A case report and review of the literature. Nutrition & Metabolism, 6(1), 10.

Miller, A. H., & Raison, C. L. (2016). The role of inflammation in depression: From evolutionary imperative to modern treatment target. Nature Reviews Immunology, 16(1), 22–34.

Samsel, A., & Seneff, S. (2013). Glyphosate's suppression of cytochrome P450 enzymes and amino acid biosynthesis by the gut microbiome: Pathways to modern diseases. Entropy, 15(4), 1416–1463.

Sarris, J., et al. (2015). Nutritional medicine as mainstream in psychiatry. The Lancet Psychiatry, 2(3), 271–274.

Simopoulos, A. P. (2016). An increase in the omega-6/omega-3 fatty acid ratio increases the risk for obesity. Nutrients, 8(3), 128.

CHAPTER 7

How Blood Sugar Influences Mental Health

——

"Blood sugar control is fundamental to mood stability. Chronic blood sugar spikes and crashes may worsen mood swings and contribute to the onset or exacerbation of depression." – Dr Georgia Ede, nutritional psychiatrist and mental health specialist

Stable blood sugar levels are essential for maintaining consistent moods, cognitive clarity, and energy – all necessary elements in mental health recovery. Dysregulated blood sugar can significantly exacerbate symptoms of depression and anxiety (Lassale et al., 2019). Blood sugar fluctuations are especially impactful for those recovering from trauma, as the stress hormone cortisol, which is often elevated in trauma survivors, can lead to significant blood sugar spikes. The pages ahead cover the connections between blood sugar balance and mental health, providing strategies for managing blood sugar to support strength and health.

The Blood Sugar-Stress Cycle: The Role of Cortisol

When stress triggers the hypothalamic-pituitary-adrenal (HPA) axis, cortisol is released, raising blood sugar to fuel the body's "fight-or-flight" response. Although this response is adaptive for short-term stress, chronic cortisol elevation – often a consequence of unresolved trauma or prolonged stress – causes frequent blood sugar imbalances, increasing cravings, mood swings, and fatigue. These fluctuations may significantly amplify anxiety, reducing emotional resilience and stability (Noble et al., 2017).

Chronic stress also makes the body less responsive to insulin, increasing the likelihood of insulin resistance. This not only affects physical health but also contributes to mood instability, irritability, and cognitive fatigue, complicating mental health recovery. By managing blood sugar, individuals can mitigate these cycles of cortisol-induced blood sugar imbalances, building a sense of calm and stability.

How Blood Sugar Dysregulation Affects Mental Health

Blood Sugar Spikes and Crashes

Consuming high-sugar foods results in rapid blood sugar spikes, followed by abrupt drops, which often lead to fatigue, irritability, and cravings – worsening symptoms of depression and anxiety. In a 2017 study, individuals consuming diets high in refined sugars had an increased risk of developing mood disorders, reinforcing the impact of diet on mental health (Knüppel et al., 2017).

Insulin Resistance and Depression

Repeated blood sugar spikes can lead to insulin resistance, a state where cells become less responsive to insulin. This condition has been shown to increase the likelihood of depression by approximately 60% (Pan et al., 2011). This is particularly concerning for individuals recovering from trauma, as chronic stress often results in elevated blood sugar levels, intensifying mental health challenges.

Hypoglycaemia (Low Blood Sugar)

Episodes of low blood sugar, or hypoglycaemia, trigger symptoms such as shakiness, anxiety, irritability, and brain fog. Studies have shown that low blood sugar levels increase irritability and are associated with higher risks of mental health disturbances (Riby, 2004). Keeping blood sugar levels stable can help reduce these symptoms, building a greater sense of mental and emotional stability.

Practical Strategies for Blood Sugar Balance

1. Balanced Meals with Protein, Fibre, and Healthy Fats

Including macronutrients like protein, fibre, and healthy fats with each meal slows down glucose absorption, promoting steady blood sugar levels. Balanced meals can reduce blood sugar spikes by up to 30% compared to high-carbohydrate meals (Jenkins et al., 2002). Key components include:

Protein: Protein slows digestion, helping maintain steady blood sugar levels.

Fibre: Fibre-rich foods, such as whole grains, vegetables, and legumes, reduce glucose absorption and minimise sugar crashes.

Healthy fats: Fats from sources like avocados, nuts, and olive oil further slow glucose release, supporting mood and energy levels.

2. Avoiding High-Sugar and Processed Foods

High-sugar and processed foods cause rapid blood sugar spikes and subsequent crashes, which destabilise mood and energy. A 2019 study highlighted that men with high sugar intake had a higher risk of developing common mental disorders (Knüppel et al., 2017). Replacing sugary foods with complex carbohydrates, like whole grains, can help improve mental clarity and reduce mood swings.

3. Regular Meal Timing

Consistent meal timing helps stabilise blood sugar levels by preventing prolonged dips and spikes. Eating every three to four hours can sustain energy levels and reduce irritability and energy crashes significantly (Jakubowicz et al., 2013). This strategy not only manages hunger but also prevents blood sugar drops that could lead to anxiety and fatigue.

4. Incorporate Magnesium and Chromium

Magnesium and chromium are essential for blood sugar regulation and insulin sensitivity. Magnesium has been shown to improve insulin sensitivity, while chromium supports cells' responsiveness to insulin (Barbagallo & Dominguez, 2010). Consuming magnesium-rich foods like leafy greens and nuts, along with chromium sources such as whole grains, can improve blood sugar control and mental clarity.

Adaptogens like ashwagandha and Rhodiola can help lower cortisol levels, supporting balanced blood sugar levels during stress. Studies indicate that adaptogens may reduce stress-related blood sugar spikes by up to 25% (Panossian & Wikman, 2010). When taken regularly, these herbs can improve emotional strength and support mental stability.

Practical Example of a Balanced Meal Plan

This meal plan example incorporates a balance of protein, fibre, and healthy fats to support blood sugar stability:

Breakfast: Greek yoghurt with berries, chia seeds, and a handful of almonds.

Lunch: Quinoa salad with mixed greens, chickpeas, and olive oil-lemon dressing.

Snack: An apple with a tablespoon of almond butter.

Dinner: Grilled salmon, roasted sweet potatoes, and steamed broccoli.

Each meal in this plan includes nutrient-dense ingredients that stabilise blood sugar, supporting mood stability and energy consistency throughout the day.

How Blood Sugar Balance Amplifies Other Healing Layers

Enhanced Mood and Energy Stability

By balancing blood sugar, individuals can experience more stable energy and reduced mood swings, which are essential for engaging in other therapies. Research suggests that blood sugar stability supports more stable mood and energy, reinforcing mental health interventions (Lassale et al., 2019).

Improved Resilience Against Stress

Controlling blood sugar levels minimises the impact of cortisol spikes, helping individuals manage stress more effectively. When blood sugar is stable, the body's reaction to stress is less severe, supporting long-term strength and mental clarity.

Reduction in Anxiety and Irritability

Balanced blood sugar reduces hypoglycaemia episodes, lowering anxiety and irritability measurably (Riby, 2004). This stability provides a solid foundation for further recovery, reducing the likelihood of mood fluctuations that can hinder progress.

Key Takeaways

Stable blood sugar reduces mood swings: Managing blood sugar helps reduce anxiety and irritability, supporting emotional stability and overall mental health.

Stress and trauma elevate blood sugar: Chronic stress leads to cortisol-induced blood sugar spikes, which contribute to emotional instability. Blood sugar control can alleviate some of these stress-related mood disturbances.

Practical dietary approaches: Prioritising balanced meals, regular meal timing, and nutrient-rich foods can bring greater mental clarity and emotional stability.

References

Barbagallo, M., & Dominguez, L. J. (2010). Magnesium and aging. Current Pharmaceutical Design, 16(7), 832–839.

Jenkins, D. J., Kendall, C. W., & Vuksan, V. (2002). Viscous fibers, health claims, and strategies to reduce cardiovascular disease risk. American Journal of Clinical Nutrition, 75(6), 1022–1033.

Jakubowicz, D., Froy, O., Wainstein, J., & Boaz, M. (2013). Meal timing and composition influence ghrelin levels, appetite scores and weight loss maintenance in overweight and obese adults. Steroids, 78(5), 615–619.

Knüppel, A., Shipley, M. J., Llewellyn, C. H., & Brunner, E. J. (2017). Sugar intake from sweet food and beverages, common mental disorder and depression: Prospective findings from the Whitehall II study. Scientific Reports, 7(1), 6287.

Lassale, C., Batty, G. D., Baghdadli, A., Jacka, F., Sánchez-Villegas, A., Kivimäki, M., & Akbaraly, T. (2019). Healthy dietary indices and risk of depressive outcomes: A systematic review and meta-analysis of observational studies. Molecular Psychiatry, 24(7), 965–986.

Noble, E. E., Hsu, T. M., & Kanoski, S. E. (2017). Gut to brain dysbiosis: Mechanisms linking Western diet consumption, the microbiome, and cognitive impairment. Frontiers in Behavioral Neuroscience, 11,

CHAPTER 8

Sunlight, Breathwork, Circadian Rhythms, and Grounding

"Exposure to sunlight, aligned with our natural circadian rhythms, coupled with conscious breathwork and grounding, can enhance mood, improve sleep, and provide the stability needed for mental health recovery."

Introduction: The Power of Natural Rhythms for Mental Health

Our bodies thrive when aligned with natural rhythms – whether through sunlight exposure, breath patterns, or direct connection with the earth's surface. These elements affect mood, sleep quality, energy levels, and emotional stability, all of which are essential for mental health. By tuning into these natural cycles, individuals can improve strength and mental clarity and reduce symptoms of depression and anxiety significantly (Riemann et al., 2012). In this chapter, we cover the interconnected benefits of sunlight exposure, circadian alignment, breathwork, and grounding practices in supporting mental health.

The Science of Circadian Rhythms and Mental Health

Circadian Rhythms: A 24-Hour Internal Clock

The body's circadian rhythm regulates sleep-wake cycles, hormone levels, energy, and mood, all of which are critical for mental health. When these rhythms are disrupted – due to irregular sleep schedules, artificial light, or lack of sunlight exposure – people may experience fatigue, irritability, and an increased risk of mood disorders. Studies show that maintaining regular circadian patterns improves strength to stress and mood stability significantly (Walker, 2017; Riemann et al., 2012).

Sunlight and Mood-Regulating Hormones

Sunlight exposure in the morning triggers serotonin production, which is essential for mood regulation and focus. Sunlight also helps regulate melatonin, the sleep hormone, which can reduce insomnia and improve sleep quality. Morning sunlight exposure has been linked to improved sleep patterns, reduced depression symptoms, and increased energy levels throughout the day (Cajochen et al., 2010; Gooley et al., 2010).

Sunlight Exposure for Mental Health

Vitamin D Synthesis and Its Impact on Mood

Sunlight exposure helps vitamin D production, which is critical for brain health and mood stability. Low vitamin D levels have been linked to increased symptoms of depression and anxiety, with studies indicating that adequate sunlight exposure can reduce depressive symptoms significantly (Bertone-Johnson et al., 2012; Holick, 2007).

Seasonal Affective Disorder (SAD) and Light Therapy

For individuals sensitive to seasonal changes, limited sunlight in autumn and winter can exacerbate symptoms of Seasonal Affective Disorder (SAD). Light therapy, which mimics natural sunlight, has been shown to benefit 60–80% of SAD sufferers, illustrating the importance of consistent light exposure for those affected by seasonal changes (Rosenthal et al., 1984).

Practical tips for increasing sunlight exposure include:

Morning sunlight: Aim for 15-30 minutes of morning sunlight exposure to stabilise serotonin levels and support melatonin production for better sleep.

Outdoor activities: Incorporate outdoor activities like walking or exercising outside, which can improve energy and mood meaningfully.

Light therapy for limited sunlight: For those in low-light climates, light therapy boxes can provide similar benefits, helping to align circadian rhythms.

Breathwork as a Tool for Mental Clarity and Emotional Resilience

Breathwork, or structured breathing techniques, can reduce stress, improve focus, and enhance emotional strength. Regular breathwork practice has been shown to reduce symptoms of anxiety and improve mental clarity (Brown & Gerbarg, 2005).

The physiological effects of breathwork on mental health include:

Regulating the autonomic nervous system: Slow, deep breathing activates the vagus nerve, which engages the parasympathetic nervous system, fostering relaxation and reducing cortisol levels.

Increasing oxygen flow to the brain: Breathwork improves oxygenation, supporting cognitive function, focus, and overall mental clarity.

Balancing Heart Rate Variability (HRV): Techniques like box breathing and alternate nostril breathing improve HRV, which is associated with reduced anxiety and greater strength to stress (Sarkar et al., 2015).

Effective breathwork techniques include:

Box breathing: Inhale for a count of four seconds, hold for four, exhale for four, and hold for four. This technique reduces anxiety and improves focus.

4-7-8 breathing: Inhale for a count of four seconds, hold for seven, and exhale for eight. This method calms the mind and is particularly effective before sleep.

Alternate nostril breathing: This practice, or Nadi Shodhana, balances the body's energy flow, improving cognitive function and reducing stress (Pramanik et al., 2009).

Grounding: Connection with the Earth for Mental Balance

Grounding, also known as earthing, involves direct physical contact with the earth, such as walking barefoot on grass, soil, or sand, which allows for the transfer of free electrons from the earth into the body. Research suggests that grounding may reduce inflammation, lower cortisol, and promote mental clarity, supporting stress resilience and emotional stability (Chevalier et al., 2012; Oschman et al., 2015).

The science says that grounding can:

Reduce inflammation: Grounding neutralises free radicals, reducing oxidative stress and inflammation – both factors associated with mood disorders.

Calm the nervous system: Grounding is thought to reduce nervous system reactivity by balancing electrical charges, leading to a calmer mental state.

Support circadian rhythms: Some studies suggest that grounding may help regulate sleep-wake cycles, particularly for those who experience jet lag or sleep disruptions.

Some practical tips for incorporating grounding include:

Daily outdoor time: To help with grounding, spend 10-20 minutes each day barefoot on natural surfaces like grass, soil, or sand.

Grounding mats: For those in urban areas or with limited outdoor access, grounding mats can simulate contact with the earth's surface.

Combine with breathwork: Practising deep breathing while grounding outdoors can improve relaxation and support mental clarity.

Amplifying Healing with Sunlight, Breathwork, and Grounding

Improved Sleep Quality

Sunlight exposure, breathwork, and grounding all contribute to high-quality sleep by aligning circadian rhythms, reducing anxiety, and decreasing inflammation. Enhanced sleep quality supports mood stability and strength, amplifying the benefits of other therapeutic layers significantly (Walker, 2017).

Enhanced Focus and Energy

Breathwork improves focus and mental clarity, while sunlight and grounding reduce fatigue and stabilise energy. Together, these practices provide an additional boost to daily cognitive function and strength (Brown & Gerbarg, 2005).

Reduced Inflammation and Emotional Resilience

Lowering cortisol through breathwork and grounding reduces systemic inflammation, a contributor to depressive symptoms. The cumulative effect promotes cognitive health and supports mental clarity, reinforcing a solid foundation for mental health (Miller & Raison, 2016).

Key Takeaways

Natural rhythms as a foundation for recovery: Aligning with circadian rhythms, sunlight exposure, breathwork, and grounding reduce depressive symptoms and support emotional strength.

Layered approach to sunlight, breathwork, and grounding: Combining these practices amplifies mood stability, reduces stress, and improves cognitive function.

Amplification of other layers: Sunlight, breathwork, and grounding improve sleep, reduce inflammation, and stabilise energy, strengthening the combined healing approach.

Next Steps

Prioritise morning sunlight: Aim for 15-30 minutes of morning sunlight each day to support serotonin and melatonin balance.

Incorporate breathwork practices: Begin with daily box breathing or 4-7-8 breathing for anxiety relief and focus enhancement.

Practice grounding regularly: Spend 10-20 minutes daily connecting with the earth, either through barefoot time outside or grounding mats indoors.

References

Bertone-Johnson, E. R., Powers, S. I., Spangler, L., et al. (2012). Vitamin D intake and depression in postmenopausal women: A large prospective study. American Journal of Epidemiology, 176(11), 1043–1050.

Brown, R. P., & Gerbarg, P. L. (2005). Sudarshan Kriya yogic breathing in the treatment of stress, anxiety, and depression: Part I – neurophysiologic model. Journal of Alternative and Complementary Medicine, 11(1), 189–201.

Cajochen, C., et al. (2010). Evening exposure to LED-backlit computer screens affects circadian physiology and sleep behaviour. Journal of Applied Physiology, 110(5), 1432–1438.

Chevalier, G., Sinatra, S. T., Oschman, J. L., Delany, R. M., & Ventura, C. (2012). Earthing (grounding) the human body reduces blood viscosity – a major factor in the grounding practice. Journal of Alternative and Complementary Medicine, 18(3), 229–237.

Gooley, J. J., et al. (2010). Exposure to room light before bedtime suppresses melatonin onset and shortens melatonin duration in humans. Journal of Clinical Endocrinology & Metabolism, 95(3), 1194–1200.

Holick, M. F. (2007). Vitamin D deficiency. New England Journal of Medicine, 357(3), 266–281.

Miller, A. H., & Raison, C. L. (2016). The role of inflammation in depression: From evolutionary imperative to modern treatment target. Nature Reviews Immunology, 16(1), 22–34.

Oschman, J. L., Chevalier, G., & Brown, R. (2015). The effects of grounding (earthing) on inflammation, the immune response, wound healing, and prevention and treatment of chronic inflammatory and autoimmune diseases. Journal of Inflammation Research, 8, 83–96.

Pramanik, T., Sharma, H., Mishra, S., et al. (2009). Immediate effect of slow pace bhastrika pranayama on blood pressure and heart rate. Journal of Alternative and Complementary Medicine, 15(3), 293–295.

Riemann, D., et al. (2012). The circadian system and sleep in depression and anxiety. Dialogues in Clinical Neuroscience, 14(4), 445–453.

Rosenthal, N. E., et al. (1984). Seasonal affective disorder and light therapy. Archives of General Psychiatry, 41(1), 72–80.

Sarkar, S., et al. (2015). Heart rate variability in psychiatry. Indian Journal of Psychiatry, 57(4), 401–405.

Walker, M. P. (2017). Why We Sleep: Unlocking the power of sleep and dreams. Scribner.

CHAPTER 9

Why Environmental Detox Matters for Mental Health

"The science is clear: Healthy buildings are foundational to a healthy workforce. Air quality, lighting, and other environmental factors are tied to improved cognitive function, better mood, and enhanced productivity." – Dr Joseph Allen, co-author of Healthy Buildings: How indoor spaces drive performance and productivity

Introduction: The Link Between Environmental Detox and Mental Health

Our environments have a profound effect on our health, especially mental health. Factors such as air quality, carbon dioxide (CO_2) levels, heavy metals, and natural sunlight exposure influence mood, cognition, and strength. Intentional environmental detoxification – reducing exposure to pollutants and increasing sunlight – can improve mood, mental clarity, and resilience significantly (Allen et al., 2016; Cajochen et al., 2010). This chapter covers the practical benefits of creating a healthier environment as a significant component in mental health recovery.

Key Environmental Factors That Impact Mental Health

Indoor Air Quality and CO_2 Levels

Indoor air quality directly affects cognitive function, mood, and energy levels. In poorly ventilated spaces, high CO_2 levels can lead to cognitive impairment, fatigue, and irritability. Research shows that reducing indoor CO_2 levels and improving ventilation can improve cognitive task performance scores by 61–101%, helping to boost mental clarity and focus (Allen et al., 2016).

Improve ventilation: Open windows regularly and use exhaust fans to improve airflow and reduce CO_2 levels.

Air purifiers and fresh air breaks: HEPA filters and regular outdoor breaks provide an additional layer of support, lowering pollutant levels indoors.

Exposure to Natural Sunlight

Natural sunlight plays a vital role in regulating circadian rhythms, which in turn affects mood, sleep, and strength. Sunlight exposure is critical for vitamin D production, which is essential for brain health. Studies show that regular sunlight exposure can reduce depressive symptoms and improve sleep quality, contributing to emotional stability (Cajochen et al., 2010; Young, 2007).

Morning sunlight: Aim for 15-30 minutes of morning sunlight to support mood regulation and melatonin production for better sleep.

Daily sunlight breaks: Incorporate sunlight breaks, particularly in winter, to compensate for lower light exposure and support mental clarity.

Heavy Metals and Neurotoxins

Heavy metals like lead and mercury disrupt brain function, cognition, and mood regulation. Chronic exposure to these metals – often found in certain foods, water, and household items – can result in mood instability and cognitive impairment. Reducing exposure to heavy metals through filtered water, minimising high-mercury fish, and using toxin-free products may improve mood stability and clarity significantly (Grandjean & Landrigan, 2014).

Filter drinking water: Use a water filter to reduce exposure to heavy metals and other contaminants in tap water.

Choose low-mercury foods: Avoid seafood with high mercury levels, such as swordfish and tuna, and opt for lower-mercury options like salmon or shrimp.

Household Cleaners and VOCs

Many household cleaners release volatile organic compounds (VOCs), which can worsen respiratory issues, fatigue, and mood swings. VOCs, common in cleaning products and air fresheners, contribute to indoor air pollution, negatively impacting both physical and mental health. Using natural or fragrance-free cleaning products reduces VOC exposure, potentially supporting mood stability (Rudel et al., 2016).

Switch to natural cleaning solutions with fewer harmful chemicals, or make DIY cleaners using ingredients like vinegar and baking soda.

Strategies for Optimising Your Environment

Improve Indoor Air Quality and CO_2 Levels

Maintaining clean indoor air is foundational for mental clarity and strength, as it helps regulate CO_2 levels and reduces exposure to pollutants.

Increase ventilation: Open windows or use exhaust fans to improve airflow, which can meaningfully enhance cognitive performance.

Take fresh air breaks: Step outside for brief breaks to lower CO_2 exposure and enhance mood.

Use indoor plants and air purifiers: Certain plants, like spider plants and peace lilies, are particularly good at absorbing CO_2, helping to clean the air. HEPA filters remove airborne particles, further supporting mental clarity.

Increase Sunlight Exposure

Exposure to natural light, especially in the morning, is one of the simplest ways to support circadian rhythms and promote mood stability.

Morning sunlight: Start the day with 15-20 minutes of sunlight exposure to help regulate circadian rhythms, reduce depressive symptoms substantially, and improve mental strength (Cajochen et al., 2010).

Daily sunlight breaks: Aim for regular outdoor time to counteract limited indoor lighting, particularly in winter.

Vitamin D supplementation: If daily sunlight is insufficient, consider vitamin D supplements to support brain health. These supplements could potentially improve mood and strength (Young, 2007).

Reduce Exposure to Household Chemicals and Heavy Metals

Toxins from household cleaners and metals in drinking water can accumulate in the body over time, affecting mental health.

Opt for natural cleaners: Use products free from VOCs to reduce respiratory issues and stabilise mood.

Filter drinking water: Install a filter to reduce heavy metal exposure, improving mental clarity and reducing cognitive impairment (Grandjean & Landrigan, 2014).

Minimise plastic use: Reduce plastic in food storage to avoid endocrine disruptors like BPA, which affect hormone balance and mood stability.

How Environmental Detoxification and Sunlight Exposure Amplify Other Healing Layers

Enhanced Mood and Cognitive Clarity

Clean air, lower CO_2 levels, and sunlight exposure support mental clarity and strength, with a cumulative boost (Allen et al., 2016). This environmental support helps people engage better in therapeutic activities, improving insight retention and focus.

Improved Sleep and Circadian Rhythm Regulation

Exposure to natural light and reduction of indoor pollutants support circadian rhythm alignment, improving sleep quality. High-quality sleep improves mood stability and strength, creating a solid foundation for sustained mental health (Cajochen et al., 2010).

Increased Motivation and Physical Energy

Regular exposure to sunlight and fresh air not only boosts mental health but also supports physical health. This combination can improve motivation and energy, leading to an enhancement in daily mental and physical well-being (Young, 2007).

Reduced Inflammatory Load

Reducing exposure to environmental toxins lowers systemic inflammation, strengthening stress resilience and emotional stability. This reduction in inflammation complements other layers in the healing process, such as diet and sleep, reinforcing a holistic approach to mental health (Rudel et al., 2016).

Key Takeaways

Environmental detox and sunlight as foundations: Optimising air quality, reducing CO_2, and increasing sunlight exposure improve mental clarity and strength.

Focus on air and sunlight exposure: By targeting indoor air quality and natural light exposure, individuals can stabilise mood and cognitive function, creating a solid base for further healing.

Amplification of other layers: These environmental adjustments reinforce sleep, diet, and therapy benefits, adding cumulative improvements for holistic mental health recovery.

Next Steps

Optimise air quality and CO_2 levels: Use air purifiers, ventilate indoor spaces, and incorporate indoor plants to improve cognitive clarity.

Increase sunlight exposure: Make sunlight exposure part of your daily routine, aiming for improvements in mood stability and circadian regulation.

Reduce chemical and heavy metal exposure: Replace household cleaners with natural alternatives, use water filters, and minimise plastic to reduce neurotoxic exposure and improve mental clarity.

References

Allen, J. G., et al. (2016). Associations of cognitive function scores with carbon dioxide, ventilation, and volatile organic compound exposures in office workers. Environmental Health Perspectives, 124(6), 805–812.

Cajochen, C., et al. (2010). Evening exposure to LED-backlit computer screens affects circadian physiology and sleep behavior. Journal of Applied Physiology, 110(5), 1432–1438.

Grandjean, P., & Landrigan, P. J. (2014). Neurobehavioral effects of developmental toxicity. The Lancet Neurology, 13(3), 330–338.

Rudel, R. A., et al. (2016). Food packaging and bisphenol A and bis(2-ethylhexyl) phthalate exposure: Findings from a dietary intervention. Environmental Health Perspectives, 119(7), 914–920.

Young, S. N. (2007). How to increase serotonin in the human brain without drugs. Journal of Psychiatry and Neuroscience, 32(6), 394–399.

CHAPTER 10

Why Gut Health Matters for Mental Wellness

"Depression is not just in the mind; it's deeply rooted in the body, with the gut playing a key role in driving the inflammation that affects how we feel emotionally." – Dr Emeran Mayer, The Mind-Gut Connection

"The gut and brain are deeply interconnected, influencing each other through a complex network that impacts everything from mood to cognitive clarity."

Introduction: The Gut-Brain Connection and Mental Health

The gut-brain connection, known as the "gut-brain axis", is increasingly recognised for its profound impact on mood, mental clarity, and strength to stress. At the heart of this connection is the gut microbiome – the diverse community of bacteria, fungi, and other microorganisms residing in the digestive tract. This microbiome plays an important role in producing neurotransmitters, managing inflammation, and regulating the body's stress response. Research shows that improving gut health can lead to improvements in mental clarity, emotional stability, and resilience, making it an essential component of mental health recovery (Dinan & Cryan, 2017; Foster & Neufeld, 2013).

The Science of the Gut-Brain Axis

Neurotransmitter Production and Regulation

Although approximately 90% of the body's serotonin is produced in the gut, this peripheral serotonin does not appear to cross the blood–brain barrier. Its relevance to mood is therefore likely indirect — via effects on gut signalling, immune activity, vagal nerve pathways, and tryptophan metabolism. Beneficial gut bacteria also help synthesise gamma-aminobutyric acid (GABA) and dopamine, which are essential for stress strength and emotional stability. Supporting a balanced microbiome may yield 15–25% improvements in mood and stress stability by promoting neurotransmitter production and regulation (Sudo et al., 2004; Carabotti et al., 2015).

Inflammation and the Gut-Brain Connection

Dysbiosis, or an imbalance in the microbiome, can elevate systemic inflammation – a key contributor to mood disorders such as depression and anxiety. High levels of pro-inflammatory cytokines are linked to worsened mood and cognitive function. A 2025 systematic review in Gut Microbiome linked decreased gut microbial diversity to greater depression symptoms, identifying specific alterations: increased abundance of pro-inflammatory genera within the Pseudomonadota phylum and decreased abundance of beneficial, short-chain fatty acid-producing Bacillota (such as Faecalibacterium) are closely associated with depressive and anxiety phenotypes. Addressing gut health with anti-inflammatory foods, probiotics, and lifestyle changes can reduce these inflammatory markers and support mood recovery.

Short-Chain Fatty Acids (SCFAs) and Brain Health

Beneficial gut bacteria produce short-chain fatty acids (SCFAs) like butyrate, acetate, and propionate, which support brain health by reducing inflammation and reinforcing the blood-brain barrier. Increased SCFA production may enhance cognitive function, emotional strength, and neuroplasticity (Dalile et al., 2019).

The Gut's Influence on the Hypothalamic-Pituitary-Adrenal (HPA) Axis

The HPA axis, central to the body's stress response, can be dysregulated due to dysbiosis, resulting in an amplified stress response. A balanced gut microbiome positively influences the HPA axis, reducing stress reactivity and providing a boost in strength and emotional stability (Sudo et al., 2004).

Understanding Risk Factors for Microbiome Imbalance

Certain life factors can predispose individuals to microbiome imbalances, which may affect mental health over time. For instance, individuals born via C-section may lack some of the beneficial bacteria typically transferred during vaginal birth. Additionally, frequent antibiotic use, particularly multiple rounds within a single year, can disrupt microbiome diversity. Studies indicate that multiple rounds of antibiotics can increase the risk of depression and anxiety, likely due to reduced bacterial diversity and increased inflammation in the gut (Lurie et al., 2015).

These factors highlight the importance of proactive microbiome support for those with higher risk profiles, such as incorporating prebiotic and probiotic-rich foods and lifestyle practices that encourage a balanced microbiome. Consulting with a healthcare professional can also be valuable for understanding and addressing specific microbiome challenges.

Dietary and Lifestyle Strategies for Supporting Gut Health

Emphasise Fresh, Whole Foods with Protein and Healthy Fats

A diet rich in fresh, minimally processed foods provides essential nutrients that support both gut and mental health. Whole foods such as vegetables, fruits, lean proteins, and healthy fats help create a balanced gut microbiome, stabilise blood sugar, and provide sustained energy.

Protein sources: Lean meats, fish, eggs, legumes, and high-quality plant-based proteins aid neurotransmitter production and support mood stability.

Healthy fats: Avocado, olive oil, nuts, seeds, and fatty fish reduce inflammation and help sustain energy, improving gut balance and resilience.

Increase Dietary Fibre and Prebiotic Foods

Prebiotics, found in fibre-rich foods, feed beneficial gut bacteria, improving microbiome diversity and stability. Fresh sources of prebiotics, such as bananas, oats, apples, and asparagus, provide fibre that supports a healthier microbiome and may yield improvements in mental clarity and mood (Dinan & Cryan, 2017; Gibson et al., 2017).

Incorporate Probiotic-Rich Foods

Probiotics, found in fermented foods like yoghurt, kefir, sauerkraut, and kimchi, introduce beneficial bacteria into the gut, helping restore balance. Consistent probiotic intake can improve mood stability and mental clarity, with benefits typically emerging within two to four weeks, especially when paired with prebiotic fibre (Sarkar et al., 2016).

Polyphenol-Rich Foods for Microbial Diversity

Polyphenols, abundant in foods such as berries, green tea, dark chocolate, and olive oil, support beneficial bacterial growth and reduce inflammation. Consuming polyphenol-rich foods regularly can support gut diversity and support mood and strength (Vauzour et al., 2015).

Additional Approaches to Supporting Gut Health

Intermittent Fasting and Gut Health

Intermittent fasting, which involves alternating periods of eating and fasting, can improve gut health by promoting beneficial bacterial diversity and supporting cellular repair processes within the digestive tract. Regular fasting may strengthen gut health and mental clarity by enhancing microbial balance and reducing inflammation (de Cabo & Mattson, 2019).

Sunlight Exposure on the Abdomen

Exposure to natural sunlight on the abdomen may improve gut health by supporting vitamin D synthesis, which supports immune function and microbial diversity. Sunlight exposure on the abdomen, especially in the morning, can further support gut and mental health by improving microbial health and reducing inflammation (Holick, 2011).

Exploring Microbiome Testing Options

In recent years, various microbiome tests have become available, providing detailed profiles of gut bacterial composition. These tests can be valuable tools for understanding specific imbalances or gut health concerns. However, interpreting microbiome results is complex and requires expertise. It's essential to consult a professional who can guide you in understanding the results and in creating a personalised plan based on the findings. By working with a knowledgeable practitioner, you can ensure the insights from microbiome testing effectively support your mental wellness journey.

How Gut Health Amplifies Other Healing Layers

Enhanced Mood Stability and Cognitive Clarity

A balanced microbiome supports neurotransmitter production and reduces inflammation, leading to improvements in mood stability, strength, and cognitive function. This creates a foundation that improves the effects of sleep, diet, and therapy (Carabotti et al., 2015).

Better Emotional Regulation and Stress Resilience

A healthy microbiome supports SCFA production and HPA axis regulation, which strengthen stress resilience and emotional stability (Dalile et al., 2019).

Improved Sleep Quality and Circadian Rhythm Regulation

The gut microbiome's influence on serotonin production also affects melatonin levels and sleep quality. Enhanced sleep due to a healthy gut may add to mental clarity and emotional well-being (Benedict et al., 2016).

Reduced Inflammatory Load Across Systems

A balanced gut microbiome lowers systemic inflammation, supporting brain health and reducing depressive symptoms. This reduction in inflammation amplifies the benefits of diet, sleep, and therapeutic practices, contributing to better mental health outcomes (Miller & Raison, 2016).

Key Takeaways

Gut health as a core component of recovery: Optimising gut health can independently and meaningfully improve mental health, providing a foundation for strength and stability.

Support the microbiome with targeted diet and lifestyle choices: Emphasise fresh, whole foods with adequate protein and healthy fats, prebiotics, probiotics, and polyphenol-rich foods while minimising disruptors.

Amplification of other healing layers: A balanced microbiome improves mood regulation, cognitive function, and inflammation reduction, strengthening the combined healing approach.

Next Steps

Add fresh, fibre-rich, and prebiotic foods: Include foods like bananas, oats, and berries to support beneficial bacteria, aiming for improvements in mental strength.

Incorporate probiotics and psychobiotics: Consume probiotic-rich foods like yoghurt and consider psychobiotic supplements to support gut-brain communication, aiming for improvement in mood stability.

Prioritise sleep and stress management: Engage in sleep-enhancing practices and stress reduction, supporting gut health and mental clarity.

References

Benedict, C., Vogel, H., Jonas, W., Woting, A., Blaut, M., Schürmann, A., & Cedernaes, J. (2016). Gut microbiota and sleep: A bidirectional relationship. European Journal of Clinical Nutrition, 70(7), 864–870.

Carabotti, M., Scirocco, A., Maselli, M. A., & Severi, C. (2015). The gut-brain axis: Interactions between enteric microbiota, central and enteric nervous systems. Annals of Gastroenterology, 28(2), 203–209.

Cajochen, C., Frey, S., Anders, D., Späti, J., Bues, M., Pross, A., & Stefani, O. (2010). Evening exposure to LED-backlit computer screens affects circadian physiology and sleep behavior. Journal of Applied Physiology, 110(5), 1432–1438.

Dalile, B., Van Oudenhove, L., Vervliet, B., & Verbeke, K. (2019). The role of short-chain fatty acids in microbiota-gut-brain communication. Nature Reviews Gastroenterology & Hepatology, 16(8), 461–478. https://doi.org/10.1038/s41575-019-0157-3

Dinan, T. G., & Cryan, J. F. (2017). Gut-brain axis in 2016: Brain-gut-microbiota axis – Mood, metabolism, and behaviour. Nature Reviews Gastroenterology & Hepatology, 14(2), 69–70.

Foster, J. A., & McVey Neufeld, K. A. (2013). Gut-brain axis: How the microbiome influences anxiety and depression. Trends in Neurosciences, 36(5), 305–312.

https://doi.org/10.1016/j.tins.2013.01.005

Gibson, G. R., Hutkins, R., Sanders, M. E., Prescott, S. L., Reimer, R. A., Salminen, S. J., ... & Reid, G. (2017). The International Scientific Association for Probiotics and Prebiotics (ISAPP) consensus statement on the definition and scope of prebiotics. Nature Reviews Gastroenterology & Hepatology, 14(8), 491–502.

Hamblin, M. R. (2017). Mechanisms and applications of the anti-inflammatory effects of photobiomodulation. APL Bioengineering, 1(1), 011002.

Holick, M. F. (2011). Vitamin D: A d-lightful solution for health. Journal of Investigative Medicine, 59(6), 872–880.

Lurie, I., Yang, Y. X., Haynes, K., Mamtani, R., & Boursi, B. (2015). Antibiotic exposure and the risk for depression, anxiety, and psychosis: A population-based study. JAMA Psychiatry, 72(9), 822–829.

Miller, A. H., & Raison, C. L. (2016). The role of inflammation in depression: From evolutionary imperative to modern treatment target. Nature Reviews Immunology, 16(1), 22–34.

Monda, V., Villano, I., Messina, A., Valenzano, A., Esposito, T., Moscatelli, F., ... & Monda, M. (2017). Exercise modifies the gut microbiota with positive health effects. Oxidative Medicine and Cellular Longevity, 2017, Article 3831972.

Sarkar, A., Lehto, S. M., Harty, S., & Dinan, T. G. (2016). Psychobiotics and the manipulation of bacteria-gut-brain signals. Trends in Neurosciences, 39(11), 763–781.

Sudo, N., Chida, Y., Aiba, Y., Sonoda, J., Oyama, N., Yu, X. N., ... & Koga, Y. (2004). Postnatal microbial colonization programs the HPA system for stress response in mice. The Journal of Physiology, 558(1), 263–275.

Tomova, A., Bukovsky, I., Rembert, E., Yonas, W., Alwarith, J., Barnard, N. D., & Kahleova, H. (2019). The effects of a plant-based diet on biomarkers of inflammation and environmental toxins in children with obesity: A randomized controlled trial. Nutrients, 11(9), 1933.

Vauzour, D., Rodriguez-Mateos, A., Corona, G., Oruna-Concha, M. J., & Spencer, J. P. E. (2015). Polyphenols and human health: Prevention of disease and mechanisms of action. Nutrients, 2(11), 1106–1131. https://doi.org/10.3390/nu7021106

CHAPTER 11

Discovering the Right Psychotherapy for Your Recovery

Introduction: Addressing Depression Through Trauma-Informed Therapy

Depression often arises from complex interactions of unresolved trauma, cognitive patterns, and physical responses stored in the body. Many people with depression have tried only one type of therapy, sometimes finding limited success when a more integrated approach could offer better results. Selecting the right treatment or combination of therapies is important to sustainable healing. "Top-down therapies" (e.g., Cognitive Behavioural Therapy (CBT), Acceptance and Commitment Therapy (ACT)) target thoughts and beliefs, while "bottom-up therapies" (e.g., Somatic Experiencing (SE), EMDR) address trauma stored in the body. This chapter introduces methods to assess your personal therapeutic needs and provides guidance on selecting approaches to create a comprehensive, trauma-informed pathway to mental health.

Identifying Your Therapeutic Approach: Top-Down vs. Bottom-Up

Choosing between top-down and bottom-up therapies depends on your unique mental health profile. For some, depression is influenced by deep-seated cognitive beliefs, while others may experience symptoms rooted in the body's responses to trauma. The following self-assessment tools can help clarify which therapeutic approach may be most effective for you.

Using Assessments to Guide Your Therapy

Adverse Childhood Experiences (ACE) Questionnaire

- Purpose: The ACE questionnaire assesses exposure to traumatic events in childhood. A higher score indicates increased exposure to trauma, which can affect physical and mental health in adulthood.
- Recommendation: Individuals with high ACE scores may benefit from bottom-up therapies to help address the physical aspects of trauma, as the body may retain trauma responses that cognitive therapy alone may not fully resolve.

Depression Anxiety Stress Scales (DASS-21)

- Purpose: Measures levels of depression, anxiety, and stress. Elevated scores in these areas provide insight into which aspects of mental health are most pressing.
- Recommendation: High anxiety and stress scores may suggest a heightened level of physiological arousal, which body-based therapies can help calm. However, if depression scores are high without significant stress or anxiety, top-down approaches like CBT may be particularly useful for addressing negative thought patterns.

Post-traumatic Stress Disorder Checklist for DSM-5 (PCL-5)

- Purpose: The PCL-5 assesses PTSD symptoms, including re-experiencing, avoidance, and hyperarousal. A high score suggests trauma symptoms that may benefit from bottom-up therapies such as EMDR and Somatic Experiencing.

- Recommendation: Scores on the PCL-5 can indicate whether trauma-focused therapy is needed, helping guide individuals to therapies that directly address trauma's physical and emotional components.

> *Note: If both ACE and PCL-5 scores are high, consider a primary focus on bottom-up therapies, which address trauma held in the body. For those with primarily cognitive symptoms on the DASS-21, top-down approaches may be more beneficial, initially.*

Top-Down Therapy Approaches and Their Benefits

Overview: Top-down therapies engage the prefrontal cortex, focusing on altering thought patterns to influence emotional and behavioural responses. These therapies are highly effective for managing cognitive symptoms of depression and anxiety.

Cognitive Behavioural Therapy (CBT)

- Efficacy: CBT is shown to reduce depressive symptoms by up to 60% over 12–20 sessions, with long-term benefits sustained through skill practice (Hofmann et al., 2012).

- Core techniques:

- Cognitive restructuring: Identifying and reframing negative thoughts that reinforce depressive feelings.

- Behavioural activation: Encouraging engagement in enjoyable or productive activities to counter depressive withdrawal.

- Thought-stopping: Techniques to interrupt negative thought cycles.
- Suggested plan: 12–20 weekly sessions, with the potential for periodic maintenance sessions for ongoing support.

Acceptance and Commitment Therapy (ACT)

- Efficacy: ACT supports strength and cognitive flexibility. Studies have shown a 40-50% reduction in depressive symptoms over 10–12 sessions (Hayes et al., 2012).
- Core techniques:
- Cognitive defusion: Observing thoughts without attachment reduces their emotional impact.
- Mindfulness: Fostering present-moment awareness and acceptance of challenging emotions.
- Values-based goals: Focusing on actions aligned with personal values to create a sense of purpose.
- Suggested plan: 10–12 weekly sessions, with emphasis on building skills for long-term application.

Dialectical Behaviour Therapy (DBT)

- Efficacy: Originally developed for borderline personality disorder, DBT is effective in helping individuals regulate intense emotions, often showing a 30-50% improvement in emotional stability over 24–30 weeks (Linehan, 1993).
- Core techniques:
- Emotion regulation: Skills for managing and processing strong emotions.
- Distress Tolerance: Techniques to endure distressing situations without impulsive reactions.
- Mindfulness: Developing non-judgemental awareness of emotional states.

- Suggested plan: DBT is often structured as a six-month programme, including weekly individual and group sessions, and is beneficial for individuals with heightened emotional sensitivity.

Bottom-Up Therapy Approaches and Their Benefits

Overview: Bottom-up therapies focus on regulating the autonomic nervous system, which stores responses to trauma. By working with the body's physiological reactions, these therapies provide relief from physical manifestations of trauma and reduce emotional distress.

Somatic Experiencing (SE)

- Efficacy: SE reduces trauma symptoms by resolving stored physical tension, which is shown to improve emotional regulation and decrease PTSD symptoms (Payne et al., 2015).
- Core techniques:
- Body scanning: Identifies areas of tension, fostering awareness of physical sensations linked to trauma.
- Titration: Processing trauma in small increments to avoid overwhelming emotional responses.
- Grounding exercises: Helps individuals feel connected to their bodies and present in the moment.
- Suggested plan: 10–20 sessions, beginning weekly, then transitioning to bi-weekly as stability improves.

Eye Movement Desensitisation and Reprocessing (EMDR)

- Efficacy: EMDR significantly reduces trauma-related depression, with studies showing 50% or more symptom reduction after 6–12 sessions (Shapiro, 2001).

- Core techniques:

- Bilateral stimulation: Uses eye movements or tactile cues to reprocess traumatic memories.

- Resource installation: Reinforces strength by focusing on positive beliefs during sessions.

- Safe place visualisation: Helps create a mental space of safety, reducing anxiety during processing.

- Suggested plan: 6–12 weekly sessions for most trauma cases, although complex trauma may require additional sessions.

Additional Therapies: Brainspotting, Clayfield Therapy, and Family Constellation Therapy

Brainspotting

- Overview: Brainspotting identifies specific eye positions linked to unprocessed trauma, allowing for targeted emotional release.

- Suggested plan: Typically, 8–15 sessions, depending on the severity and complexity of the trauma.

Clayfield Therapy

- Overview: Uses tactile interaction with clay to externalise trauma, allowing individuals to confront and reshape memories safely.

- Suggested plan: 10–15 weekly sessions.

Family Constellation Therapy

- Overview: Focuses on inherited patterns from family trauma, using group or individual role-playing to resolve family dynamics.

- Suggested plan: One to three initial sessions, with follow-ups every few months as needed.

Practical Applications for Combining Top-Down and Bottom-Up Therapies

- The following steps outline a practical approach to gradually integrating top-down and bottom-up therapies into a combined, layered practice:
- Awareness: Begin with mindfulness and cognitive restructuring to understand thought patterns and triggers.
- Adding Body-Based Techniques: Gradually incorporate grounding or body scanning to connect mental and physical awareness.
- Building Routine: Balance cognitive and body-based techniques throughout the week to reinforce resilience.
- Case Examples:
- CBT with Somatic Experiencing: Cognitive restructuring is paired with somatic techniques, allowing individuals to address mental and physical symptoms simultaneously.
- EMDR with Grounding Techniques: Safe place visualisations and grounding exercises improve EMDR sessions, creating a secure foundation for processing trauma.

Daily Routine Suggestions

- Morning: Start with mindfulness meditation or breathing exercises to centre and prepare for the day.
- Afternoon: Use cognitive tools, such as journaling or thought records, to assess and reframe thoughts.
- Evening: Practice body-based techniques like progressive muscle relaxation or body scanning to release tension.

Amplified Benefits of Combining Top-Down and Bottom-Up Approaches

- Enhanced self-awareness and emotional regulation: Top-down therapies support cognitive awareness, while bottom-up therapies stabilise the body's responses, creating emotional balance.
- Strengthened mind-body connection: Combining cognitive and body-based methods improves the integration of mind and body, supporting whole-person healing.
- Increased strength and flexibility: A combined approach strengthens strength, making it easier to manage future stressors and prevent relapse.

References

Beck, A. T. (2016). Cognitive therapy: Nature and relation to behaviour therapy. Behavioral Therapy, 1(2), 184–200.

Berceli, D., & Napoli, M. (2006). A proposal for body-oriented trauma intervention training for first responders. International Journal of Emergency Mental Health, 8(4), 275–287.

Courtois, C. A., & Ford, J. D. (2009). Treating Complex Traumatic Stress Disorders: An evidence-based guide. Guilford Press.

Hayes, S. C., Strosahl, K. D., & Wilson, K. G. (2012). Acceptance and Commitment Therapy: The process and practice of mindful change. Guilford Press.

Hofmann, S. G., Asnaani, A., Vonk, I. J., Sawyer, A. T., & Fang, A. (2012). The efficacy of cognitive behavioral therapy: A review of meta-analyses. Cognitive Therapy and Research, 36(5), 427–440.

Karatzias, T., et al. (2021). Polyvagal Theory and trauma treatment: An evidence-based review. Frontiers in Psychology, 12, 678–689.

Lee, C. W., & Cuijpers, P. (2013). A meta-analysis of the contribution of eye movements in processing emotional memories. Journal of Behavior

Therapy and Experimental Psychiatry, 44(2), 231–239.

Levine, P. A. (2010). In An Unspoken Voice: How the body releases trauma and restores goodness. North Atlantic Books.

Linehan, M. M. (1993). Cognitive-behavioral Treatment of Borderline Personality Disorder. Guilford Press.

Payne, P., Levine, P. A., & Crane-Godreau, M. A. (2015). Somatic experiencing: Using interoception and proprioception as core elements of trauma therapy. Frontiers in Psychology, 6, 93.

Porges, S. W. (2009). The Polyvagal Theory: Neurophysiological foundations of emotions, attachment, communication, and self-regulation. Norton & Company.

Resick, P. A., Monson, C. M., & Chard, K. M. (2016). Cognitive Processing Therapy for PTSD: A thorough manual. Guilford Press.

Shapiro, F. (2001). Eye Movement Desensitization and Reprocessing: Basic principles, protocols, and procedures. Guilford Press.

van der Kolk, B. A. (2014). The Body Keeps the Score: Brain, mind, and body in the healing of trauma. Viking.

CHAPTER 12

Memory as a Foundation for Healing

Introduction: The Role of Memory in Mental Health

Memory is central to our sense of self, shaping how we view life experiences and ourselves. Autobiographical memories, which are typically coherent and reflective, help us learn, grow, and create a stable self-narrative. In contrast, traumatic memories are often fragmented and sensory-based, making them harder to integrate into our life stories. For people recovering from depression, balancing these memory types can build strength, mental clarity, and emotional stability. The focus here is on how understanding and integrating memories – both autobiographical and traumatic – can improve mental health recovery.

The Science of Autobiographical and Traumatic Memory

1. Autobiographical Memory: Reflection and Self-Understanding

Autobiographical memory is the coherent recall of life events, typically processed in the brain's prefrontal cortex, which supports organised thinking and reflection. These memories allow people to connect past experiences in a balanced way, reinforcing a positive and stable sense of self.

Individuals with depression often experience disruptions in positive autobiographical memory recall, leading to a self-narrative skewed toward negative experiences. Techniques that encourage recalling positive memories help rebuild a balanced self-narrative, supporting strength and clarity (Dalgleish & Werner-Seidler, 2014).

2. Traumatic Memory: Sensory-Based and Fragmented Experiences

Traumatic memories are stored differently. Instead of coherent recollection, they often remain in a fragmented form, relived through sensory fragments – like sounds, sensations, or visuals – that make it hard to move past the trauma. This phenomenon, known as "sensorimotor fragmentation", keeps traumatic memories vivid and often intrusive, leading to heightened anxiety and mood dysregulation.

The amygdala, responsible for emotional responses, becomes hyperactive during trauma, encoding memories in a way that bypasses typical cognitive organisation. This can result in a constant sense of threat, making people feel they are re-experiencing trauma rather than recalling it. Dr Ruth Lanius' research highlights how these disorganised memories affect emotional regulation and increase the need for therapies that facilitate trauma integration (Lanius et al., 2010).

Therapeutic Approaches for Memory Integration

Top-Down Therapies for Autobiographical Memory Reframing

- Cognitive Behavioural Therapy (CBT):
- Research and efficacy: CBT is widely recognised for helping reframe negative autobiographical memories, with studies showing up to a 60% reduction in depressive symptoms (Beck, 2016).

- Applications: Techniques such as cognitive restructuring and positive memory recall promote a more balanced self-narrative, enhancing self-esteem and emotional stability.
- Acceptance and Commitment Therapy (ACT):
- Overview: ACT encourages acceptance of challenging thoughts and feelings, improving cognitive flexibility and mindfulness. Research shows that ACT can reduce depressive symptoms by approximately 40-50% (Hayes et al., 2012).
- Applications: By building present-moment awareness and a values-based approach, ACT supports self-identity and purpose, helping people to build a self-narrative based on growth and strength.
- Narrative Therapy:
- Overview: Narrative therapy involves re-authoring one's life story, allowing individuals to view their past with empowerment and objectivity. This externalises challenges, helping to reframe experiences as part of a larger, meaningful life story.
- Applications: Developing a constructive, empowered narrative helps individuals contextualise their experiences positively, strengthening self-identity and strength.
- Internal Family Systems (IFS):
- Overview: IFS explores internal "parts" of oneself – such as protective or vulnerable aspects – to build inner balance. It supports understanding and resolution of internal conflicts that often arise after traumatic experiences.
- Applications: By working with internalised emotions or dialogues, IFS enables the integration of self-narratives and supports emotional harmony.

Bottom-Up Therapies for Trauma and Somatic Memory Integration

- Brainspotting:

- Overview: Brainspotting uses eye positioning to access deep-seated trauma within the brain, allowing targeted release and emotional relief.

- Efficacy: Studies show that Brainspotting can be especially helpful for trauma that other therapies have not resolved. It involves accessing hidden memories through focused eye positions.

- Applications: Brainspotting connects trauma's sensory aspects to present awareness, integrating fragmented memory into a cohesive narrative.

- Clayfield Therapy:

- Overview: This somatic-based therapy allows individuals to mould traumatic memories into physical shapes, enabling tactile processing of trauma.

- Applications: Modelling memories with clay externalises emotions, helping safe confrontation and release, which is especially beneficial for those struggling to express trauma verbally.

- Family Constellation Therapy:

- Overview: This therapy examines inherited trauma patterns in family dynamics, often using group or individual role-playing to explore and resolve generational issues.

- Efficacy: Effective for individuals affected by family trauma or unresolved relational patterns, Family Constellation Therapy allows people to observe familial influences objectively.

- Applications: By reenacting family roles, individuals gain insight into how inherited trauma impacts their lives, enabling emotional release and self-distancing from these patterns.

Building a Balanced Memory Narrative

1. Recognising and Shifting Negative Memory Biases

In depression, people often focus on negative memories, reinforcing feelings of hopelessness. Recognising and rebalancing this bias by emphasising positive memories is essential. Techniques such as gratitude journaling and positive memory recall help redirect the brain's focus toward constructive memories, creating strength against depressive thought patterns.

2. Promoting Positive Memory Recall

Therapies that emphasise recalling positive experiences can combat depressive thought patterns and enhance mental strength. Techniques like savouring or visualising joyful memories provide a foundation of positive autobiographical memories that buffer against negativity.

How Memory Integration Amplifies Other Healing Layers

1. Enhanced Emotional Regulation

Integrating and processing traumatic memories reduces emotional intensity, leading to improved emotional stability. This stability makes it easier to engage with other therapies, like mindfulness or cognitive restructuring and builds a strong mindset.

2. Improved Cognitive Flexibility

Memory integration helps reduce negative biases and fosters cognitive flexibility, enabling individuals to reinterpret experiences more constructively. This flexibility improves their ability to approach life challenges with a positive outlook, supporting a growth-oriented perspective.

3. Nervous System Reset and Physical Health Benefits

Trauma often keeps the sympathetic nervous system "stuck" in a heightened state of fight-or-flight, which can disrupt gut health, hormone regulation, and emotional strength. Bottom-up therapies, such as Somatic Experiencing and Sensorimotor Psychotherapy, work directly on the body's responses, releasing stored physical tension and calming the nervous system. This reset supports gut health, hormonal balance, and overall healing, aligning the mind and body for whole-person recovery.

4. Strengthened Self-Identity and Purpose

Balancing and integrating traumatic and autobiographical memories reinforces a coherent self-narrative. This stable self-identity allows individuals to engage in positive relationships, pursue meaningful goals, and approach life with a sense of purpose and confidence.

Key Takeaways

- Memory processing as a foundation for healing: Understanding how autobiographical and traumatic memories influence mental health provides insight into tailored therapeutic approaches.
- Addressing negative memory biases: Rebalancing negative memory biases supports a stable self-narrative and strength,

reducing depressive symptoms.

- Diverse approaches for memory integration: Integrative therapies like Brainspotting, Family Constellation Therapy, and Narrative Therapy offer innovative ways to address both trauma and autobiographical memory, amplifying strength, mental clarity, and emotional health.

References

Beck, A. T. (2016). Cognitive Therapy: Nature and relation to behavior therapy. Behavioral Therapy, 1(2), 184–200.

Dalgleish, T., & Werner-Seidler, A. (2014). Memory in depression: Twenty years of research. Psychological Medicine, 44(4), 789–795.

Hayes, S. C., Strosahl, K. D., & Wilson, K. G. (2012). Acceptance and Commitment Therapy: The process and practice of mindful change. Guilford Press.

Lanius, R. A., et al. (2010). The nature of traumatic memories: A speculative approach. Clinical Psychology Review, 30(2), 126–135.

Ogden, P., & Fisher, J. (2015). Sensorimotor Psychotherapy: Interventions for trauma and attachment. W. W. Norton & Company.

Shapiro, F. (2001). Eye Movement Desensitization and Reprocessing: Basic principles, protocols, and procedures. Guilford Press.

Williams, J. M. G., et al. (2007). Autobiographical memory specificity and emotional disorder. Psychological Bulletin, 133(1), 122–148.

CHAPTER 13

Digital Detox and Media Consumption

Introduction: Understanding the Digital Impact on Mental Health

In today's fast-paced, tech-focused world, constant digital engagement has become the norm. While technology offers numerous benefits, excessive screen time and social media consumption can negatively impact mental health, contributing to heightened stress, disrupted sleep, and difficulty focusing. This chapter introduces the concept of a digital detox, aimed not at removing technology entirely but at creating a balanced digital environment that supports mental well-being. By making intentional choices around digital use, you can reduce stress, enhance focus, and improve sleep quality – all of which are foundational for combined healing.

The Effects of Excessive Digital Consumption

Recent research has explored the impact of digital media use on mental health, finding that high levels of screen time, particularly on social media, can increase anxiety, lower self-esteem, and interfere with sleep patterns (Sun, 2023;

Marciano et al., 2022). Additionally, findings suggest that, while smartphones and social media use do not directly cause mental health problems, how we interact with digital media – and our awareness of its impact on health – can be key (Odgers, 2024). By adopting mindful digital habits, you can create a healthier relationship with technology that supports a calm and focused mind.

Doomscrolling and the Negative News Cycle

One of the most common digital habits that negatively affects mental health, especially in individuals experiencing depression, is doomscrolling – endlessly consuming negative news, often from a 24-hour news cycle. Constant exposure to distressing news stories can create a cycle of fear and negativity, increasing stress, anxiety, and feelings of helplessness. For those recovering from depression, this can reinforce pessimistic thoughts and disrupt emotional balance, as research indicates that exposure to negative news can fuel symptoms of depression and anxiety (Viner et al., 2019).

To counter this, consider limiting news consumption to a specific time each day, perhaps from reputable sources known for balanced reporting. Curating a healthier news diet allows you to stay informed without overwhelming your mental health, contributing to a more positive and stable emotional state.

Digital Hygiene Checklist

Use this checklist to develop healthier, more intentional digital habits that support your mental health goals.

- Turn off notifications: Constant notifications pull your attention away from the present moment, increasing stress and reducing focus. You can adjust your device settings to turn off non-essential notifications, such as app alerts, email notifications, and social media notifications.

- Set daily screen limits: Monitoring and limiting screen time helps you become more aware of how much time you spend online. Many devices have built-in screen-time trackers. Set daily limits for apps that you find especially consuming, such as social media or news platforms.

- Unfollow negative influences: The content you consume directly impacts your mood and outlook. Review your social media feeds and unfollow accounts that promote negativity, stress, or comparison. Focus on following people and pages that inspire and uplift you.

- Incorporate screen-free times: Designate specific times in your day as screen-free, especially in the evening before bed. To improve sleep quality, avoid screens for at least an hour before bed. Blue light from devices can interfere with the body's natural sleep rhythm (Chang et al., 2015).

- Use "do not disturb" mode: Enabling "do not disturb" mode during focused activities helps you stay present without interruptions. Experiment with scheduling "do not disturb" times during work, family meals, or any activity where you want to be fully engaged.

- Limit social media checks: Social media can be a significant source of stress, particularly with constant checking. Try limiting social media checks to a few times a day and logging out of apps after each session. This will help you stick to your designated times.

- Curate your content: Be intentional about the type of content you consume. Subscribe to newsletters, podcasts, and media that provide positive and educational content. This helps counteract the tendency for digital spaces to fill with overwhelming or negative information.

The Benefits of a Digital Detox for Mental Health

Reducing screen time and practising digital hygiene can offer significant mental health benefits:

- Reduced stress and anxiety: Limiting notifications and social media can reduce the constant influx of information and pressure to respond, which can lower stress (Hoge et al., 2017).
- Improved sleep: Minimising screen use before bed helps your body align with its natural circadian rhythm, promoting better sleep. Good sleep is essential for mental health recovery, as it supports mood regulation and energy levels (Cain & Gradisar, 2010).
- Enhanced focus and productivity: Reducing screen time frees up mental bandwidth, improving concentration and reducing mental fatigue. This can lead to higher productivity and a more focused mind (Rosen et al., 2013).
- Increased emotional strength: Curating your digital content to include positive influences can counterbalance the stress and comparison often associated with social media. By creating a supportive digital environment, you create a mental space that fosters resilience and positivity (Przybylski & Weinstein, 2017).

Using Technology Wisely: Evidence-Based Mental Health Apps

While reducing passive and distressing digital consumption is important, technology can also be a positive tool in depression recovery when used intentionally. A 2025 meta-analysis in the Journal of Medical Internet Research, examining 18 randomised controlled trials involving 3,477 participants, confirmed that AI-driven conversational therapy apps produce reliable reductions in depressive symptoms, with 30–51% symptom improvement in mild-to-moderate depression (Drissi et al., 2025). Apps such as Sleepio (CBT-I focused) and Woebot (CBT based) have the strongest RCT evidence.

One important caveat: AI therapy apps consistently perform below the level of a human therapist (who achieve 45–50% improvement on average) and are not a substitute for professional care in moderate-to-severe depression. They are most valuable as a starting point while waiting for a therapist, as a between-session supplement to existing therapy, or as a maintenance tool during periods of relative stability – not as a replacement for the real thing.

Practical Steps for a Gradual Digital Detox

Here are some practical steps to ease into a digital detox, gradually creating lasting changes in your digital habits:

- Start small: Begin by choosing one or two items from the digital hygiene checklist and focus on them for a week. For instance, set a daily screen limit or designate a screen-free time in the evening.

- Reflect on changes: After a week, reflect on any shifts in mood, focus, and sleep quality. Noticing the positive impact can reinforce the benefits of balanced digital habits.

- Build your digital boundaries gradually: As you feel comfortable, add more elements from the checklist, such as unfollowing negative influences or turning off notifications.
- Schedule a regular digital detox day: Choose one day each week to stay offline or significantly reduce screen time. This break from constant engagement can help refresh your mind and give you a much-needed digital pause.

Conclusion: A Balanced Digital Life for Mental Wellness

Creating a balanced digital life can significantly improve one's mental well-being. By practising digital hygiene and making intentional choices about screen time, one creates an environment that builds focus, peace, and positivity. A digital detox isn't about removing technology but about finding a balance that supports one's layered healing journey. With each step, one reclaims mental space and clarity, which is essential for sustained mental health.

References

Andreassen, C. S., Griffiths, M. D., Gjertsen, S. R., Krossbakken, E., Kvam, S., & Pallesen, S. (2013). The relationships between behavioural addictions and the five-factor model of personality. Journal of Behavioral Addictions, 2(2), 90–99.

Cain, N., & Gradisar, M. (2010). Electronic media use and sleep in school-aged children and adolescents: A review. Sleep Medicine, 11(8), 735–742.

Chang, A.-M., Aeschbach, D., Duffy, J. F., & Czeisler, C. A. (2015). Evening use of light-emitting eReaders negatively affects sleep, circadian timing, and next-morning alertness. Proceedings of the National Academy of Sciences, 112(4), 1232–1237.

Hoge, E., Bickham, D., & Cantor, J. (2017). Digital media, anxiety, and depression in children. Pediatrics, 140(2), S76-S80.

Marciano, L., Ostroumova, M., Schulz, P. J., & Camerini, A.-L. (2022). Digital media use and adolescents' mental health during the Covid-19 pandemic: A systematic review and meta-analysis. Frontiers in Public Health, 9, Article 793868.

Odgers, C. L. (2024). The panic over smartphones doesn't help teens. The Atlantic. Retrieved from https://www.theatlantic.com/technolog y/archive/2024/05/candice-odgers-teens-smartphones/678433

Przybylski, A. K., & Weinstein, N. (2017). A large-scale test of the Goldilocks hypothesis: Quantifying the relations between digital-screen use and the mental health of adolescents. Psychological Science, 28(2), 204–215.

Drissi, N., Ouhbi, S., Janati Idrissi, M. A., & Fernandez-Luque, L. (2025). Effectiveness of AI-driven conversational agents in improving mental health among young people: Systematic review and meta-analysis. Journal of Medical Internet Research, 27, e69639. https://doi.org/10.2196/69639

Rosen, L. D., Carrier, L. M., & Cheever, N. A. (2013). Facebook and texting made me do it: Media-induced task-switching while studying. Computers in Human Behavior, 29(3), 948–958.

Sun, L. (2023). Social media usage and students' social anxiety, loneliness and health: Does digital mindfulness-based intervention effectively work? BMC Psychology, 11, Article 362.

Tudehope, L., Harris, N., Vorage, L., & Sofija, E. (2024). What methods are used to examine representation of mental ill-health on social media? A systematic review. BMC Psychology, 12, Article 105.

Twenge, J. M., & Campbell, W. K. (2018). Associations between screen time and lower psychological well-being among children and adolescents: Evidence from a population-based study. Preventive Medicine Reports, 12, 271–283.

Viner, R. M., Gireesh, A., Stiglic, N., Hudson, L. D., Goddings, A. L., Ward, J. L., & Nicholls, D. E. (2019). Roles of cyberbullying, sleep, and physical activity in associations between social media use and mental health in young people: A systematic review. The Lancet Child & Adolescent Health, 3(10), 685–696.

CHAPTER 14

Beyond the Therapy Session – Living Your Psychotherapy Skills

Introduction: Embedding Therapy Skills in Daily Life for Sustainable Healing

The true power of therapy is realised when it becomes part of daily life. Moving beyond weekly sessions to integrate grounding, cognitive restructuring, and self-compassion into your daily routine fosters strength, laying a solid base for other health practices like sleep, nutrition, and physical activity. Let's look at how to practice therapeutic skills consistently, creating layers that support emotional regulation, physical health, and mental clarity for a whole-person, sustainable recovery.

Integrating Therapy Skills into Everyday Routines

1. Daily Practice of Therapy Techniques for Emotional Stability

Integrating therapeutic techniques into each part of the day creates a consistent emotional foundation, amplifying the benefits of other practices.

- Morning routine: Begin with grounding practices such as deep breathing, gratitude journaling, or affirmations. These calm the nervous system, anchoring you for the day ahead and reducing emotional reactivity. This foundation complements physical movement, aligning with practices from Chapter 8 on circadian rhythm, sunlight, and grounding, which improve mood and energy.

- Midday check-in: Practicing cognitive restructuring in the middle of the day prevents stress from escalating. Skills from CBT and ACT (discussed in Chapter 11) help reframe negative thoughts, improve focus and stabilise mood. Pairing cognitive techniques with mindful eating, as noted in Chapter 7 on blood sugar, stabilises energy levels and reinforces mental clarity.

- Evening reflection: Ending with gratitude journaling or positive memory recall helps calm the mind for restful sleep, supporting practices from Chapter 4 on sleep optimisation. Integrating reflection with sleep hygiene routines reduces cortisol levels, improving sleep quality and mood stability.

2. Developing Self-Awareness and Emotional Regulation

Developing self-awareness strengthens emotional regulation, which supports additional healing layers such as physical health, social support, and mindfulness.

- Identifying patterns and triggers: Daily journaling or mood tracking highlights emotional patterns and reveals triggers, as discussed in Chapter 12 on memory integration. Recognising these patterns creates a proactive buffer against triggers, reducing their impact on hormone balance and gut health, as explored in Chapter 9.

- Practising distress tolerance and grounding: Techniques like distress tolerance from DBT and grounding exercises stabilise emotional responses. As discussed in Chapter 10, body-based approaches calm the sympathetic nervous system, improving overall resilience and aligning with gut and hormone regulation.

- Self-compassion practices: Self-compassion exercises, like self-kindness affirmations, reduce self-criticism and build strength. Self-compassion integrates with grounding practices, providing a foundation for stability that complements both self-care and mindfulness routines.

Relapse Prevention and Sustained Recovery through Layered Assessment and Support

Consistent self-assessment and a strong support network build accountability and strength, reinforcing combined healing.

1. Routine Self-Assessment

- Monthly check-in with DASS-21 and other assessments: Using tools like the DASS-21 or PCL-5, as outlined in Chapter 10, provides valuable insight into progress, highlighting areas that may need additional focus. Routine assessments create structure, lowering relapse risk and improving the stability of other therapeutic layers.
- Daily mood and goal tracking: Tracking mood and setting small daily goals helps maintain awareness of mental health patterns and strengthens a sense of progress. This daily tracking strengthens connections between mood, diet, and sleep (explored in Chapters 4, 5, and 6), offering a thorough view of how lifestyle choices influence mental well-being.

2. Building a Robust Support System

A strong support network of family, friends, and therapeutic resources amplifies emotional resilience, adding accountability and community to the healing layers.

- Social support from family and friends: Building trusted relationships builds motivation, accountability, and encouragement. Strong social support reduces the risk of relapse by creating emotional stability and enhancing overall recovery, which is essential for engaging in regular physical activity, as described in Chapter 5.

- Therapeutic maintenance check-ins: Regular check-ins with a therapist reinforce skills and offer tailored support for new challenges. Consistent therapeutic guidance stabilises emotional regulation and supports layers like daily self-care and strength techniques.

- Peer support groups: Peer networks provide shared experience, empathy, and encouragement. Structured peer support improves strength and adds accountability, validating the healing process and strengthening the emotional and social support layers.

Integrating Other Healing Layers for Comprehensive Recovery

Therapy skills create a base that amplifies additional layers of healing, such as physical health, mindfulness, and structured routines, forming a comprehensive approach to recovery.

1. Physical Health as a Core Layer

- Nutrition and movement: Consistent exercise and a diet rich in anti-inflammatory foods reduce inflammation, increase energy, and support emotional resilience. As explored in Chapters 4 and 5, aligning physical health practices with emotional stability promotes recovery from both mental and physical perspectives.

- Sleep hygiene for restoration: As discussed in Chapter 3, quality sleep strengthens mood stability and cognitive clarity, forming a solid bedrock for mental health. Pairing sleep hygiene practices with evening therapy skills supports restful sleep and reinforces the benefits of emotional regulation techniques.
- Mindfulness and relaxation practices: Mindfulness and relaxation exercises reduce stress and improve strength. As noted in Chapter 8, practices like meditation, yoga, and body scans align seamlessly with therapy skills, creating a balanced, strong core for emotional and physical well-being.

2. Integrative Healing Practices for Ongoing Support

Integrative therapies, such as red light therapy, aromatherapy, or neuroacoustic sound therapy, offer targeted support, reducing stress and supporting calm. These methods reinforce mental clarity and stability, improving the effects of therapy skills by creating a balanced environment for sustainable recovery.

How Layering Amplifies Recovery

Layering therapeutic practices throughout the day creates a cumulative effect where each routine, habit, and practice reinforces the next, leading to sustainable strength and recovery.

- Emotional layering: Consistent use of skills like grounding, cognitive restructuring, and self-compassion builds a reliable emotional foundation, which allows for the addition of complementary practices like mindfulness or distress tolerance.

- Physical layering: Adding physical health routines, such as nutrition, exercise, and sleep, stabilises mood and energy and amplifies the effects of mental health practices. This combined approach creates a feedback loop between mind and body that improves strength.

- Social and community layering: Establishing social support through family, friends, and peer groups reinforces therapeutic layers, creating accountability, reducing isolation, and adding relational stability to the recovery journey.

Key Takeaways

- Daily integration of therapy skills: Practicing therapeutic skills consistently builds emotional stability, reducing stress and relapse risk by up to 60% (Hofmann et al., 2012).

- Layering physical, emotional, and social supports: Physical health, emotional awareness, and social connection reinforce each other, creating a stable and supportive environment for long-term healing.

- Comprehensive lifestyle integration: By combining therapy skills with lifestyle practices, such as nutrition, sleep hygiene, and mindfulness, individuals build physical, mental, and emotional strength and foster lasting recovery.

References

Emmons, R. A., & McCullough, M. E. (2003). Counting blessings versus burdens: An experimental investigation of gratitude and subjective well-being in daily life. Journal of Personality and Social Psychology, 84(2), 377–389.

Fava, G. A., et al. (2004). Relapse prevention in unipolar depression: Cognitive behavioral strategies after remission of acute depressive episodes. Psychotherapy and Psychosomatics, 73(5), 249–254.

Hofmann, S. G., et al. (2012). The efficacy of cognitive behavioral therapy: A review of meta-analyses. Cognitive Therapy and Research, 36(5), 427–440.

Irwin, M. R. (2015). Why sleep is important for health: A psychoneuroimmunology perspective. Annual Review of Psychology, 66, 143–172.

Kabat-Zinn, J. (1990). Full Catastrophe Living: Using the wisdom of your body and mind to face stress, pain, and illness. Delacorte Press.

Lakey, B., & Orehek, E. (2011). Relational regulation theory: A new approach to explain the link between perceived social support and mental health. Psychological Review, 118(3), 482–495.

Neff, K. D. (2011). Self-compassion: The proven power of being kind to yourself. William Morrow.

Sarris, J., et al. (2015). Nutritional medicine as mainstream in psychiatry. The Lancet Psychiatry, 2(3), 271–274.

Wichers, M., et al. (2011). Daily life moment-to-moment variability in depressed and remitted individuals: Reduced complexity and variability. Psychological Medicine, 41(3), 467–476.

Yalom, I. D., & Leszcz, M. (2005). The Theory and Practice of Group Psychotherapy. Basic Books.

CHAPTER 15

Psychoneuroimmunology and the Healing Power of Creativity, Laughter, and New Interests

"The immune system responds not only to our physical environment but to our perceptions and beliefs as well. When we live with emotions of joy, creativity, and connection, our immune system responds by strengthening our defences. When we live in fear, resentment, or isolation, our physiology follows." – Dr Mario Martinez

Introduction: Psychoneuroimmunology – The Connection Between Mind, Body, and Immunity

Psychoneuroimmunology (PNI) is the scientific study of the interplay between the mind, emotions, the immune system, and overall health. Research has shown that our mental and emotional states can profoundly impact immune health, demonstrating how joy, laughter, creativity, and social connection bolster strength, mental clarity, and physical defences. Intentional engagement in joyful, creative, and connective activities can elevate mood, enhance immune function, and lay a supportive foundation for recovery. This chapter looks into the practical applications of PNI principles and shows how a combined approach can be used to reinforce both mental and physical wellness.

The Science of Psychoneuroimmunology: How Mental States Affect Physical Health

1. Immune Responses and Emotional States

Positive emotions like joy, gratitude, and connection have significant impacts on immune function. Emotions shape immune responses, as positivity lowers inflammatory markers and boosts immune cell activity. Research demonstrates that laughter reduces cortisol and stimulates natural killer cell production, helping fight infections and chronic illness. For instance, laughter therapy has been shown to decrease stress by 20-40% and increase immune markers, supporting physical strength (Bennett et al., 2003).

2. Creativity and Neurotransmitter Release

Engaging in creative activities, like painting, music, and writing, stimulates dopamine release, a neurotransmitter associated with motivation, pleasure, and reduced stress. Creative expression strengthens neural pathways, supports cognitive flexibility, and can decrease cortisol levels by up to 30% (Forgeard et al., 2014). Regular creative activities positively influence mental health, supporting strength when combined with physical health practices.

3. Social Connection and Immunity

Engaging in social activities – such as group singing, communal art projects, or community sports – improves immune function by increasing oxytocin levels, a hormone associated with trust and connection. Studies reveal that social solid bonds lower inflammation, improve immune responses, and increase strength to stress (Cohen, 2004). Integrating social activities with other foundational layers, like regular movement and mindfulness, amplifies emotional and physical benefits, reinforcing well-being.

Healing Through Joy and Creativity

Laughter as Medicine

Laughter stimulates the release of endorphins and serotonin, alleviating stress and creating a sense of health. Known for its pain-relieving and mood-boosting effects, laughter increases strength, improves sleep, and reduces physical discomfort. Studies show that laughter lowers cortisol levels by up to 40% and significantly improves life satisfaction, with long-term benefits for immune health (Martin, 2001).

Infuse your daily life with laughter by watching comedies, listening to humorous podcasts, or recalling light-hearted memories with loved ones. A few minutes of laughter each day strengthens strength and boosts physical and mental health.

Laughter Yoga: Joy Through Movement

Laughter yoga combines intentional laughter with deep breathing exercises, creating a full-body relaxation response. The blend of laughter and movement lowers cortisol, boosts immune function, and builds a positive mindset. Laughter yoga has been shown to reduce stress hormones and increase strength. It provides a structured, joyful practice that reinforces the benefits of daily physical movement.

Try a local laughter yoga class or participate online to incorporate this unique, joyful practice. Just a few minutes daily can elevate mood, increase resilience, and improve overall immune health.

Stand-Up Comedy and Shared Laughter

Attending stand-up comedy shows or watching performances with friends offers a fun and relaxing way to experience shared laughter. This shared experience can heighten feelings of connection, relieve stress, and reinforce a sense of belonging. Research shows that shared laughter in social settings improves immune response, improves strength, and strengthens mental clarity.

Attend live stand-up comedy shows, enjoy a comedy special with friends, or even try performing at an open mic event. Stand-up comedy is an accessible, social way to reduce stress, amplify mood, and enjoy the benefits of laughter.

Expressive Arts and Freeform Creativity

Art-making without a specific goal builds relaxation, supports emotional expression, and improves focus. Studies show that regular engagement in art-making activities, such as drawing, painting, or crafting, can improve mood by up to 25% (Kaimal et al., 2016). Art also serves as a safe outlet for processing emotions, creating a foundation for strength through creative self-expression.

Dedicate time to creative projects without focusing on the outcome. Freeform creativity allows for emotional expression and can reveal underlying thoughts, helping with emotional processing and boosting mental clarity.

Singing, Music-Making, and the Vagus Nerve

Singing and music-making stimulate the vagus nerve, supporting relaxation and enhanced respiratory function. Research shows that group singing significantly lowers stress hormones, boosts immune responses, and creates feelings of connection and unity. Music engages both hemispheres of the brain, improving emotional processing, strength, and health.

Join a choir, sing along to your favourite songs, or play an instrument. These activities reduce stress, boost mood, and create a sense of community that reinforces mental and physical health.

Exploring New Hobbies and Neurogenesis

Engaging in new hobbies stimulates neurogenesis, the formation of new brain cells, supporting cognitive flexibility and improved mood. Novel experiences activate the brain's reward system, enhancing strength, satisfaction, and mental clarity. Research shows that people who regularly engage in diverse activities have improved life satisfaction, decreased anxiety, and higher stability (Heller, 2010).

Dedicate time each week to exploring new interests or hobbies, such as learning a language, trying a new sport, or starting a creative project. Consistent engagement with new activities helps prevent boredom, builds cognitive flexibility, and boosts life satisfaction.

How Creative and Joyful Activities Amplify Other Healing Layers

Enhanced Mood and Immune Function

Creative and joyful activities reduce stress hormones like cortisol, which can impair immune health. Engaging in creativity, laughter, and social connection increases serotonin and endorphins, establishing an emotional and physical environment supportive of healing. Layering these activities with foundational practices, such as nutrition (Chapter 4) and physical activity (Chapter 5), creates a combined effect, boosting strength.

Improved Social Connection and Emotional Resilience

Creativity and laughter create meaningful connections with others, which improve emotional strength and reduce the risk of anxiety and depression. Social engagement activities like group singing, art projects, or collaborative comedy nights build a sense of belonging, relieve loneliness, and support mental and physical health.

Reduced Inflammation and Physical Health Benefits

Positive emotional experiences, including laughter, creativity, and social engagement, reduce inflammatory markers, which are often elevated in chronic stress and depression. This anti-inflammatory effect helps stabilise mood, promotes long-term strength, and prevents the reoccurrence of stress-related health issues.

Integrated Mind-Body Healing through Layered Practices

Mind-body practices, such as laughter, yoga, singing, and creativity, activate the parasympathetic nervous system, calming the body and supporting immune health, gut function, and hormonal balance. Layering these practices into a thorough daily routine supports strength, stability, and long-term mental health.

Practical Guide: Layering Creativity and Joy for Enhanced Healing

- Daily laughter for immune health and strength: Daily laughter supports immune function, reduces stress, and boosts strength. Incorporating laughter through comedy shows shared jokes, or laughter yoga strengthens emotional stability and mental clarity.

- Creative outlets for emotional expression: Engaging in art, singing, or new hobbies relaxes the mind, reduces stress, and supports mood strength. These practices amplify emotional awareness, adding a foundational layer to mental and physical health.

- Building social connections through shared hobbies: Group activities, such as singing, comedy shows, or art classes, build social bonds and support immune health, improving strength across mental and physical layers.

- Creating a personal "joy prescription": Develop a personal "joy prescription" by listing activities that bring happiness and intentionally scheduling time each day to engage in them. This approach reinforces consistency, creating a combined practice that amplifies mental, physical, and emotional strength.

Key Takeaways

- Incorporate laughter into daily life: Laughter stimulates immune health, reduces stress, and boosts resilience. Integrating humour into your routine fosters a stable mental and physical state.

- Engage in creative outlets: Creative activities improve mood and mental clarity while supporting self-expression. Practices like art-making or music build strength and support physical health.

- Strengthen social bonds through shared hobbies: Group activities, such as singing, laughter yoga, or comedy nights, improve social connections, immune health, and emotional strength.

References

Bennett, M. P., et al. (2003). The effect of mirthful laughter on stress and natural killer cell activity. Alternative Therapies in Health and Medicine, 9(2), 38–45.

Cohen, S. (2004). Social relationships and health. American Psychologist, 59(8), 676–684.

Forgeard, M. J., et al. (2014). Happy people thrive: Evidence for positive emotions, subjective well-being, and psychological well-being. Journal of Positive Psychology, 9(4), 361–374.

Heller, D., et al. (2010). Beyond the "Big Five": The Big Two model and the world of personal projects. Journal of Research in Personality, 44(1), 123–137.

Irwin, M. R. (2015). Why sleep is important for health: A psychoneuroimmunology perspective. Annual Review of Psychology, 66, 143–172.

Kaimal, G., et al. (2016). Reduction of cortisol levels and participants' responses following art-making. Art Therapy, 33(2), 74–80.

Martin, R. A. (2001). Is laughter the best medicine? Humor, laughter, and physical health. Current Directions in Psychological Science, 10(6), 216–220.

Pearce, E., Launay, J., & Dunbar, R. I. M. (2016). The ice-breaker effect: Singing mediates fast social bonding. Royal Society Open Science, 3(1), 150221.

CHAPTER 16

Belief as a Healing Force

The placebo and nocebo effects reveal that beliefs and expectations significantly impact physical and mental health. When patients expect positive outcomes, they're more likely to experience tangible benefits, even from inactive treatments. Conversely, the nocebo effect can trigger negative symptoms when expectations are unfavourable. These effects highlight the profound influence of mindset on healing, a concept extensively studied in psychoneuroimmunology. Here, we examine how positive belief systems, the therapeutic alliance, and intentional practices can foster resilience and support remission from depression, amplifying the effects of both top-down and bottom-up therapies.

The Science of Placebo and Nocebo Effects

1. Placebo Effect: The Power of Positive Expectation

The placebo effect shows that when individuals expect a positive outcome, they often experience real improvements. This effect activates the brain's natural pain-relieving pathways, including the release of endorphins, dopamine, and other neurotransmitters associated with health. Studies indicate that patients who anticipate pain relief experience up to 30-40% reductions in pain perception, solely through the power of belief

(Benedetti et al., 2005). This demonstrates that mental states, particularly positive expectations, can directly influence physiological responses.

2. Nocebo Effect: The Impact of Negative Expectations

Conversely, the nocebo effect occurs when negative expectations lead to real symptoms or a worsening of conditions. Patients who anticipate side effects are more likely to experience them, even with a placebo. Research shows that negative expectations can amplify pain, discomfort, and other symptoms by up to 20-30% (Häuser et al., 2012). The nocebo effect illustrates how limiting beliefs can trigger adverse physiological responses, increasing cortisol levels and reinforcing stress.

3. The Neurobiology of Belief and Expectation

Both placebo and nocebo effects engage brain regions involved in mood, stress, and perception, including the prefrontal cortex and limbic system. Positive expectations activate the body's natural painkillers, while negative expectations stimulate stress hormones like cortisol, impacting the immune system and influencing inflammation and healing processes (Tracey, 2010). Understanding these mechanisms helps to harness belief as a healing tool, building strength through therapeutic practices and supportive relationships.

The Therapeutic Alliance and Its Influence on Outcomes

1. Therapist-Patient Relationship as a Healing Mechanism

The quality of the therapeutic alliance – the relationship between therapist and client – has a powerful impact on outcomes. When therapists express confidence in their clients' potential for recovery, they build a supportive environment that improves placebo effects, encouraging clients to believe in their capacity for healing. Studies reveal that a strong therapeutic alliance can improve patient outcomes by up to 40% across various therapies (Horvath & Symonds, 1991).

2. Limited Re-Parenting and the "Good Enough" Therapist

The concept of "limited re-parenting", where the therapist serves as a "good enough" parent, offers clients a safe, supportive relationship that addresses attachment wounds. This approach helps clients build trust, internal resources, and self-compassion. Through a dependable, validating relationship, clients reduce self-doubt and build strength, contributing to long-term improvements in mental health.

3. Setting Intentions and Fostering Positive Beliefs in Therapy

By cultivating an environment of hope, therapists help clients establish realistic, helpful beliefs about their capacity to recover. Research shows that intention-setting and positive reinforcement increase motivation, improve strength, and support the development of mental frameworks conducive to healing (Norcross & Lambert, 2018). Through intention-setting, clients build a growth-oriented mindset, reinforcing the impact of other therapeutic techniques.

Practical Strategies for Enhancing Belief and Healing in Therapy

1. Building Trust and Rapport

Creating a trustworthy environment is essential for use the placebo effect in therapy. Therapists can foster trust by using empathetic listening, validating clients' experiences, and maintaining transparency. Studies on trust and rapport show that a strong therapeutic relationship can increase treatment adherence, amplify positive expectations, and improve outcomes (Norcross & Lambert, 2018).

2. Positive Reinforcement and Validation

Positive reinforcement – acknowledging progress and celebrating small achievements – reinforces clients' belief in their progress. Consistent validation strengthens clients' expectations of success, creating a positive feedback loop that improves therapy outcomes. Clients who feel validated are more likely to engage in treatment, reinforcing a hopeful outlook.

3. Cognitive Restructuring of Negative Beliefs

Cognitive restructuring, a foundation of CBT, challenges and reframes nocebo-like expectations that may hinder progress. By addressing limiting beliefs and transforming them into constructive ones, clients reduce anxiety and adopt a positive mental framework. This shift away from self-defeating beliefs helps build strength, reinforcing a hopeful outlook and reducing vulnerability to depression.

The Therapist's Role in Psychoneuroimmunology: Fostering Physical and Emotional Healing

1. Enhancing the Client's Autonomic Balance

Therapists trained in body-based practices, such as vagus nerve stimulation, grounding exercises, or breathwork, help clients regulate their autonomic nervous systems. These techniques promote calm and balance, reducing stress responses and inflammation, which strengthens the body's natural healing capacity. Through intentional relaxation, clients support both their mental and physical health, improving therapeutic progress.

2. Promoting Self-Efficacy and Empowerment

Encouraging clients to take an active role in their healing builds a sense of control and confidence, known as self-efficacy. Studies show that a strong sense of self-efficacy is linked to reduced stress and improved immune function (Bandura, 1997). By supporting clients in setting achievable goals and taking responsibility for their recovery, therapists improve their strength, helping them develop a proactive mindset.

3. Integrating Mind-Body Techniques to Reinforce Positive Expectations

Mind-body techniques, including visualisation, breathwork, and mindfulness, reinforce positive expectations. Studies reveal that visualising positive outcomes activates the brain's reward circuits, producing physiological benefits that extend to the immune system (Kabat-Zinn, 1990). These techniques allow clients to access and sustain a hopeful mindset, amplifying the effects of therapeutic work and supporting sustained mental wellness.

How Placebo, Nocebo, and Therapeutic Alliance Amplify Other Healing Layers

1. Enhanced Mood and Immune Response

Positive expectations release dopamine and endorphins, stabilising mood and boosting immune function. Placebo effects complement top-down and bottom-up approaches, improving strength and emotional well-being. Clients who engage with therapy from a place of hope and confidence experience more effective healing, as positive expectations increase the likelihood of remission.

2. Improved Motivation and Engagement

Clients who experience strong therapeutic alliances are more motivated to engage in treatment, reinforcing the benefits of therapy, nutrition, exercise, and integrative practices. By setting small, achievable goals, and recognising progress, therapists help clients remain invested in their healing journey, creating a cumulative, combined approach to recovery.

3. Resilience to Future Stress

Building positive beliefs provides clients with tools to build strength, reducing the likelihood of relapse. As clients internalise therapeutic skills and reframe limiting beliefs, they develop a greater sense of control over their emotions and experiences. This skill set supports long-term recovery, creating a foundation for stable mental health that endures beyond therapy.

Key Takeaways

- Beliefs shape healing: Positive expectations can improve recovery, while negative beliefs can hinder it, highlighting belief as a powerful element in remission from depression.
- Therapeutic alliance as a tool: The quality of the therapist-client relationship amplifies healing outcomes, increasing the efficacy of both top-down and bottom-up therapies.
- Mind-body connection: Mind-body practices that build positive expectations improve strength, immune health, and emotional stability, providing a foundation for long-term mental wellness.

References

Bandura, A. (1997). Self-efficacy: The exercise of control. W.H. Freeman.

Benedetti, F., et al. (2005). Placebo mechanisms and the ethics of placebo use in clinical practice and research. Pain, 116(1–2), 3–6.

Häuser, W., et al. (2012). Nocebo phenomena in medicine: Their relevance in clinical practice. Deutsches Ärzteblatt International, 109(26), 459–465.

Horvath, A. O., & Symonds, B. D. (1991). Relation between working alliance and outcome in psychotherapy: A meta-analysis. Journal of Counseling Psychology, 38(2), 139–149.

Kabat-Zinn, J. (1990). Full Catastrophe Living: Using the wisdom of your body and mind to face stress, pain, and illness. Delacorte Press.

Norcross, J. C., & Lambert, M. J. (2018). Psychotherapy relationships that work: Volume 1. Oxford University Press.

Tracey, I. (2010). Placebo analgesia: Impact of psychosocial context on pain perception. Pain, 150(1), 8–10.

CHAPTER 17

Understanding the Grief Exception

Recognising Grief as Distinct from Depression

Grief and depression share overlapping symptoms – such as sadness, fatigue, and changes in appetite – but grief is typically rooted in a specific loss and involves a unique process of emotional adaptation. Unlike depression, which can persist indefinitely, grief often evolves, transitioning from acute sorrow to a more integrated acceptance. This distinction was previously acknowledged in diagnostic guidelines like the DSM-IV's Bereavement Exclusion, which advised clinicians against diagnosing major depression within the first two months of bereavement. Although this exclusion was removed in the DSM-5, it remains essential to differentiate grief from clinical depression to respect the natural process of mourning.

In this chapter, we look at the biological, emotional, and psychological differences between grief and depression and introduce approaches that respect the unique nature of grief. By understanding the distinct elements of grief, individuals can better honour their emotions and work towards healing.

The Nature of Grief and How It Differs from Depression

Biological Responses to Grief vs. Depression

Grief and depression activate different biological pathways, though both can affect mood, cognition, and energy levels. Grief involves acute stress responses, including temporary increases in cortisol, which typically subside over time as the grieving individual adapts to the loss. Depression, however, has been associated with complex neurobiological patterns, including chronic inflammation and prolonged stress hormone imbalances.

Re-evaluating the serotonin theory of depression

While the serotonin theory of depression once suggested that low serotonin levels were a primary cause of depression, recent research calls this assumption into question. An umbrella review of serotonin-related studies found no consistent link between serotonin levels and depression onset, challenging the "chemical imbalance" model. Instead, depression appears to involve multiple factors, including neurobiological, psychosocial, and environmental elements, that interact in complex ways. This evolving understanding highlights the importance of addressing depression through a complex approach rather than relying solely on serotonin-targeted treatments.

Emotional and Psychological Differences Between Grief and Depression

Grief encompasses a range of emotions, including sadness, longing, and moments of nostalgia. Unlike depression, which often brings a pervasive sense of hopelessness, grief may allow the person to recall positive memories and feel connected to the deceased loved one. Depression, however, is more likely to present as an ongoing emotional numbness or despair that is difficult to lift.

Grief may involve intense sadness but typically includes moments of peace or even joy when reminiscing about the loved one. Over time, grief tends to diminish as acceptance grows. Depression often lacks these positive emotional moments, presenting instead as an unrelenting heaviness that interferes with day-to-day functioning and persists beyond the context of any specific loss.

Recognising these emotional differences helps to validate the grieving process, allowing individuals to experience their feelings fully without conflating grief with clinical depression.

Therapeutic Approaches Unique to Grief

Grief is not a condition to be "cured", but rather an experience to be navigated and integrated. Approaches that build acceptance, honour memories, and provide space for emotional release can be particularly effective for those going through bereavement. These therapies focus on helping individuals adapt to life changes rather than minimising or avoiding their grief.

Acceptance-Based Therapies

Acceptance-based therapies, like Acceptance and Commitment Therapy (ACT), support individuals in experiencing grief without suppressing their emotions. ACT teaches acceptance of all emotions and builds resilience by helping individuals confront and process their pain with self-compassion.

ACT techniques include mindfulness exercises that allow grievers to sit with difficult emotions and accept them as part of the healing process. Mindfulness can help reduce the emotional intensity of grief, supporting a gradual adjustment to loss.

Narrative therapy enables individuals to recount memories, share stories, and explore the meaning of their loss. This form of treatment honours the deceased and helps the grieving person integrate the loss into their life narrative, providing a structured outlet for reflection and healing.

Techniques like journaling, creating memory books, or sharing stories in a therapeutic setting can comfort individuals and help them make sense of their emotions. Reflecting on the significance of the relationship can build emotional strength and acceptance.

Rituals and Commemorations

Participating in rituals or creating personal commemorations allows grievers to process their loss meaningfully. Rituals provide structure during an emotionally turbulent time and can offer a sense of closure, honouring the bond shared with the loved one.

Rituals may include visiting a loved one's resting place, lighting candles, or holding memorial ceremonies. These activities build connection, respect, and comfort, helping individuals transition from loss to remembrance.

Healing Strategies That Honour the Grieving Process

Grieving requires patience, compassion, and often a gradual re-engagement with life. Unlike depression treatment, which encourages activity and engagement, healing from grief may involve periods of solitude and reflection. Strategies that support self-compassion, social support, and emotional awareness are vital to managing grief.

Self-Compassion and Patience

Grieving individuals benefit from a gentle, compassionate approach to their emotions. Rather than pushing to "move on", they are encouraged to experience their feelings without judgement, respecting the need to grieve at their own pace.

Practicing self-compassion by acknowledging emotions without judgement and giving oneself permission to grieve openly and without time constraints.

Gradual Re-Engagement with Social Connections

While social support is essential, re-engagement should happen gradually to respect the grieving individual's need for personal space. Rebuilding connections, when ready, can provide comfort and a sense of normalcy.

Reconnecting with friends and family at a comfortable pace, through small gatherings or supportive group settings, can build connection without overwhelming the grieving person.

Mindful Reflection and Acceptance of Emotions

Mindful reflection allows individuals to observe their grief without suppressing it, encouraging a full spectrum of emotional experiences. This approach can build acceptance of complex emotions and support the grieving process without rushing it.

Engaging in mindfulness practices like meditation, breathing exercises, or journaling can help individuals process grief without avoidance, building emotional strength over time.

How Grief Support Amplifies Other Healing Layers

Grief support can improve emotional strength, social stability, and overall mental health by building a compassionate approach to healing. The following benefits show how the grieving process, when honoured, can support broader mental health recovery:

- Enhanced emotional strength and stability: Processing grief constructively builds resilience, enabling individuals to experience and accept their emotions fully. This emotional stability can create a foundation of resilience, equipping individuals with the strength to manage future challenges with greater ease.

- Improved social and relational health: As individuals process grief, they are often able to re-establish meaningful social connections with newfound empathy and perspective. This reintegration fosters healthy relationships and reduces the risks of isolation, which is important for long-term mental health.

Support for Holistic Mental Health Through Acceptance

Acceptance-based approaches, such as ACT, allow individuals to integrate grief as a natural part of their emotional landscape. This acceptance builds whole-person mental health by validating the grieving process, reducing the likelihood of unresolved grief leading to chronic emotional distress.

Key Takeaways

- Grief as a distinct emotional process: While grief and depression may appear similar, grief has unique biological and emotional components that differentiate it from clinical depression.

- Therapies that honour grief: Acceptance-based therapies, narrative therapy, and personal rituals provide supportive frameworks that respect the grieving process. They encourage emotional release without pressure to "move on".

- Holistic benefits of grieving: By supporting grief as a natural healing process, individuals are better equipped to regain emotional strength, maintain social connections, and experience mental clarity.

References

Bonanno, G. A. (2004). Loss, trauma, and human resilience: Have we underestimated the human capacity to thrive after extremely aversive events? American Psychologist, 59(1), 20–28.

Moncrieff, J., et al. (2022). The serotonin theory of depression: A systematic umbrella review of the evidence. Molecular Psychiatry, 27, 2402–2412.

Neimeyer, R. A. (2001). Meaning Reconstruction and the Experience of Loss. American Psychological Association.

Stroebe, M., Schut, H., & Stroebe, W. (2007). Health outcomes of bereavement. The Lancet, 370(9603), 1960–1973.

Worden, J. W. (2008). Grief Counseling and Grief Therapy: A handbook for the mental health practitioner. Springer Publishing.

CHAPTER 18

Rewiring the Brain for Depression Recovery – Neuroplasticity, Neurogenesis, and Brain Imaging

Leveraging Brain Imaging for Depression and Brain Injury Recovery

Depression, concussion, and traumatic brain injuries (TBI) often lead to structural and functional changes in the brain, particularly in areas involved in mood regulation, cognitive function, and resilience. Advances in brain imaging – such as WAVi, quantitative electroencephalography (qEEG), and Single Photon Emission Computed Tomography (SPECT) – allow us to visualise and track these changes, providing valuable insights into the brain's adaptation and healing process. Here we look at these technologies alongside lifestyle practices, nootropics, and advanced therapies that encourage neuroplasticity (the brain's ability to form new pathways) and neurogenesis (the growth of new neurons), creating a thorough approach to recovery from depression, TBI, and concussion.

Understanding Brain Imaging Technologies in Depression and TBI Recovery

1. WAVi (Brain Performance Assessment)

WAVi uses electroencephalography (EEG) technology to measure cognitive performance, attention, and mood metrics. Depression and TBI often correspond with reduced cognitive processing speed and attentional challenges. WAVi provides insights into underactive brain regions impacted by these conditions.

WAVi results help track improvements in cognitive processing and mood regulation as individuals engage in therapies like exercise, mindfulness, and neurofeedback. This feedback improves motivation by visually showing neuroplastic changes.

2. qEEG (Quantitative Electroencephalography)

qEEG captures and maps brainwave patterns, highlighting dysregulations associated with mood instability and cognitive difficulties. Depression, TBI, and concussions are often linked with disrupted alpha and theta waves, indicating areas in need of therapeutic intervention.

qEEG is commonly used to inform neurofeedback therapy, in which individuals train their brainwave activity to improve emotional regulation and cognitive stability. Over time, qEEG reveals improvements in brainwave coherence, helping to visualise mental stability and strength gained through therapy.

3. SPECT Imaging (Single Photon Emission Computed Tomography)

SPECT provides a detailed view of blood flow in the brain, showing areas with excessive or reduced activity. Depression and TBI may present as reduced blood flow in the prefrontal cortex and increased activity in the limbic system, both linked to mood regulation.

SPECT can guide targeted therapies, such as neurofeedback or cognitive treatment, by identifying specific brain areas needing support. Tracking changes with SPECT over time helps visualise recovery in areas impacted by TBI, depression, or concussion.

The Role of Neuroplasticity and Neurogenesis in Depression and TBI Recovery

1. Neuroplasticity: Building Resilience Through New Neural Connections

Neuroplasticity, the brain's ability to rewire and form new connections, enables the recovery of disrupted pathways in conditions like depression and TBI. By creating new neural pathways, neuroplasticity supports cognitive flexibility, emotional strength, and improved mental health.

Regular psychotherapy, including Cognitive Behavioural Therapy (CBT), Acceptance and Commitment Therapy (ACT), and Dialectical Behaviour Therapy (DBT), enhances neuroplasticity by addressing and restructuring negative thought patterns. Therapeutic exercises, such as reframing thoughts and developing new habits, help strengthen adaptive neural connections.

2. Neurogenesis: Growing New Neurons for Emotional Stability

Neurogenesis involves the growth of new neurons, primarily in the hippocampus, a region important for mood regulation and memory. Depression and TBI can impair neurogenesis, but targeted activities – like physical exercise and creative engagement – support neuronal growth, improving cognitive clarity and strength.

Aerobic exercise and creative pursuits, such as painting or writing, stimulate brain-derived neurotrophic factor (BDNF), supporting neurogenesis and supporting recovery from both depression and TBI. Studies suggest that these activities can reduce symptoms by up to 50% (Ratey & Loehr, 2011).

Advanced Therapies for Brain Healing: HBOT and Photobiomodulation

Hyperbaric Oxygen Therapy (HBOT) for Brain Repair

HBOT involves breathing pure oxygen in a pressurised chamber, increasing oxygen levels in the blood and tissues. Note that HBOT remains an emerging therapy for depression and brain injury; it is not yet a standard clinical recommendation and should be considered only under specialist medical supervision. Clinical data from 2026 confirms HBOT is particularly effective for post-stroke depression (PSD) and depression tied to ischaemic or traumatic brain injuries. A 4-week course of HBOT alleviates depressive symptoms by upregulating Brain-Derived Neurotrophic Factor (BDNF) and Nerve Growth Factor (NGF), restoring cerebral perfusion and supporting neuroplasticity.

- Key benefits: HBOT improves cellular repair, improves blood flow to damaged brain areas, and reduces inflammation, which is common after TBI. It can also improve memory, mood regulation, and cognitive function.
- Application: Treatment usually requires multiple sessions, lasting 60–90 minutes, under professional supervision.

Photobiomodulation (Red Light Therapy) for Neuroprotection and Regeneration

Photobiomodulation, or red light therapy, uses low-level red and near-infrared light to stimulate mitochondrial function in brain cells. This therapy supports neurogenesis, reduces oxidative stress, and improves blood flow, supporting recovery from TBI and improving cognitive function. A 2025 analysis in the Journal of Affective Disorders (18 trials) confirmed that PBM exerts a moderate effect in reducing depressive symptoms.

Current evidence suggests optimal parameters for transcranial application include wavelengths around 823 nm, applied for 30 minutes, 2–3 times weekly for more than 15 sessions.

- Key benefits: Red light therapy supports mitochondrial health, promotes neurogenesis, and reduces inflammation. Research shows it can improve cognitive clarity, mood stability, and emotional regulation.
- Application: Red light therapy sessions typically last 10–20 minutes and are conducted multiple times weekly. Professional guidance is recommended for optimal outcomes.

Nootropics for Neuroplasticity, Neuroprotection, and Cognitive Resilience

Creatine: Enhancing Brain Energy and Cognitive Performance

Creatine boosts brain energy by increasing ATP production, which is essential for cognitive strength and mental clarity. It is especially beneficial for those experiencing fatigue and cognitive issues post-TBI or with depressive symptoms.
Three to five grams of creatine monohydrate per day supports cognitive function and strength.

Methylene Blue: Neuroprotective and Antioxidant Effects

Methylene blue is a powerful antioxidant that supports mitochondrial health and protects neurons from oxidative damage. At low doses, it may enhance mood stability and cognitive function. However, methylene blue acts as a potent monoamine oxidase inhibitor (MAOI). Both the US FDA and the Australian TGA mandate strict boxed warnings because combining it with serotonergic psychiatric medications (such as

SSRIs, SNRIs, or TCAs) can trigger serotonin syndrome, a potentially fatal condition. It is strictly contraindicated for anyone on standard antidepressant pharmacotherapy.

Methylene blue should only be used at low therapeutic doses determined in direct consultation with a doctor. Due to the risk of fatal serotonin syndrome when combined with antidepressants including SSRIs, SNRIs, and MAOIs, do not use without medical supervision. If you are currently taking any serotonergic medication, do not use methylene blue.

Lion's Mane Mushroom and the Stamets Stack

Lion's Mane supports neurogenesis by stimulating nerve growth factor (NGF). The Stamets Stack combines Lion's Mane, niacin, and psilocybin microdoses, with large-scale observational studies reporting improvements in mood, focus, and neuroplasticity among practitioners. Because the Stamets Stack includes psilocybin — a controlled substance in Australia and many other countries — this approach must only be explored under the guidance of a qualified medical professional in a licensed clinical setting. Self-administration is not recommended and may carry legal and health risks.

Because the Stamets Stack includes psilocybin — a controlled substance in Australia and many other countries — this approach must only be explored under the guidance of a qualified medical professional in a licensed clinical setting. Self-administration is not recommended and may carry legal and health risks.

Psilocybin-Assisted Therapy: An Emerging Treatment for Treatment-Resistant Depression

Psilocybin-assisted psychotherapy represents one of the most significant advances in depression treatment in decades, particularly for treatment-resistant depression (TRD) where conventional antidepressants have not achieved remission. As of 2025, over 150 clinical trials are registered on ClinicalTrials.gov, and phase 3 trials are underway globally. A 2024 network meta-analysis confirmed that a single large dose of psilocybin (e.g., 25 mg) administered with psychological support yields rapid, substantial reductions in depressive severity. Long-term observational data shows up to 67% of participants remaining in remission for at least five years post-treatment. Australia leads internationally in this area: since July 2023, the TGA has rescheduled psilocybin (Schedule 8), allowing authorised psychiatrists to legally prescribe macro-dose psilocybin for treatment-resistant depression.

A key 2024 randomised controlled trial published in JAMA confirmed that a single carefully supervised psilocybin session produced significant reductions in depression scores that persisted for weeks to months. A subsequent network meta-analysis reported that, in closely supervised clinical trial conditions, 25 mg was associated with the strongest outcomes across depression measures (von Rotz et al., 2024). This does not constitute a dosage recommendation. The proposed mechanism involves transient disruption of the brain's default mode network, facilitating neuroplasticity, loosening rigid negative thought patterns, and supporting sustained reappraisal of past experiences.

Important context: psilocybin-assisted therapy is not yet widely approved and should only be undertaken in medically supervised clinical or licensed therapeutic settings. Self-administration is not recommended and carries significant risks. However, for individuals with treatment-resistant depression who have not responded to multiple antidepressants, discussing access to clinical trials or licensed therapy centres with a psychiatrist is a worthwhile conversation. For current availability in your country, visit clinicaltrials.gov.

Ketosis: An Alternative Fuel Source for Brain Health

Ketosis provides the brain with ketones instead of glucose, offering a more stable energy source and reducing brain fog. For individuals with depression or brain injuries, ketosis can support neuroplasticity, reduce inflammation, and improve cognitive function. The evidence base has strengthened substantially: a 2024 Stanford pilot study found that a medically supervised ketogenic diet improved psychiatric symptoms in patients with serious mental illness, with none meeting criteria for metabolic syndrome at four-month follow-up. A 2025 pilot study in college students with major depressive disorder found adding a ketogenic diet to usual care produced approximately a 69% reduction in depressive symptoms – among the largest effects seen in any dietary intervention trial (Danan et al., 2024).

A ketogenic diet or exogenous ketone supplements can help maintain stable brain energy, reduce mood fluctuations, and support cognitive clarity.

Lifestyle Pathways to Support Neuroplasticity and Brain Health

Creative Engagement and New Hobbies

Engaging in new hobbies and creative activities stimulates neuroplasticity by introducing novel cognitive challenges, promoting resilience, and improving mood stability.

Dedicate time weekly to learning new skills or engaging in creative pursuits, supporting neural connections linked to motivation and fulfilment.

Dietary Support for Brain Health

A diet rich in omega-3 fatty acids, antioxidants, and polyphenols supports neuroplasticity and neurogenesis by reducing inflammation and nourishing brain cells.

Incorporate foods like salmon, berries, leafy greens, and nuts into daily meals to enhance brain strength and reduce depressive symptoms.

Sleep and Neural Recovery

Consistent, restorative sleep is essential for neuroplasticity. It allows the brain to consolidate memories, process emotions, and repair neurons. Regular sleep also improves cognitive clarity and emotional strength.

Aim for seven to nine hours of sleep per night to support neuroplasticity, emotional balance, and cognitive health.

How Imaging Supports Neuroplasticity Practices

- Tracking neuroplastic changes: Imaging technologies like WAVi, qEEG, and SPECT provide feedback on brain changes, allowing individuals to track the effects of therapeutic interventions.

- Guiding personalised approaches: Imaging highlights specific dysregulations, allowing therapies to target areas in need of support, such as increasing blood flow or balancing brainwave patterns.

- Reinforcing motivation: Visualising tangible improvements through imaging enhances motivation, showing individuals the impact of their efforts on brain health.

Key Takeaways

- Imaging for personalised recovery: Tools like WAVi, qEEG, and SPECT enable tailored recovery plans by visualising areas affected by depression, TBI, and concussion.

- Neuroplasticity and neurogenesis as foundations for healing: Practices such as psychotherapy, exercise, and mindfulness build adaptability and restore cognitive and emotional stability.

- Advanced therapies for brain health: HBOT and red light therapy support neuroprotection and cellular repair, aiding recovery from brain injuries.

- Nootropics and ketosis for cognitive support: Creatine, methylene blue, Lion's Mane, and ketosis provide alternative sources of brain energy and protection, improving strength.

References

Beck, A. T. (2016). Cognitive therapy: Nature and relation to behavior therapy. Behavioral Therapy, 1(2), 184–200.

Gage, F. H. (2019). Neurogenesis in the adult brain. Journal of Neuroscience, 25(19), 4697–4702.

Hölzel, B. K., et al. (2011). Mindfulness practice leads to increases in regional brain grey matter density. Psychiatry Research: Neuroimaging, 191(1), 36–43.

Irwin, M. R. (2015). Why sleep is important for health: A psychoneuroimmunology perspective. Annual Review of Psychology, 66, 143–172.

Ratey, J. J., & Loehr, J. E. (2011). The positive impact of physical activity on cognition and brain function. American Journal of Lifestyle Medicine, 5(4), 335–338.

Sarris, J., et al. (2015). Nutritional medicine as mainstream in psychiatry. The Lancet Psychiatry, 2(3), 271–274.

CHAPTER 19

Building Resilience Through Connection and Community

"Connection is why we're here; it is what gives purpose and meaning to our lives." – Dr Brené Brown

Introduction: The Healing Power of Connection

Human beings are inherently social, and connection is a critical component of mental and emotional well-being. Relationships provide emotional support, accountability, and a sense of belonging that improves strength against life's challenges. Research demonstrates that social bonds can reduce depression severity by up to 50% and act as a buffer against future depressive episodes (Cohen, 2004). In this chapter, we explore the science of social connection, practical strategies for building supportive networks, and the importance of maintaining constructive focus to avoid rumination, which can hinder progress in recovery.

The Science of Social Connection and Resilience

1. Social Bonds as Protective Factors

Social connections support mental health by promoting the production of oxytocin and reducing cortisol levels, which are linked to stress and depression. Studies indicate that people with strong social ties are less likely to experience depression and anxiety. A comprehensive meta-analysis found that individuals with strong social networks have a 29% lower risk of depression and a 50% lower risk of premature mortality compared to those who are socially isolated (Holt-Lunstad et al., 2010).

Loneliness and social isolation increase the likelihood of depression by approximately 40%. Building meaningful relationships can reduce feelings of isolation and reinforce a positive sense of self, improving mental strength (Santini et al., 2020). The World Health Organization (WHO) has recognised loneliness as a global health threat. In Australia, the RACGP champions social prescribing as a formal clinical pathway.

2. Psychoneuroimmunology of Connection

Psychoneuroimmunology (PNI) explores how social interactions impact immune function, reducing inflammatory markers and improving the body's response to stress. Research has shown that individuals with strong social connections display lower levels of inflammation and higher strength, which supports improved emotional and physical health outcomes (Uchino, 2009).

Chronic loneliness and social isolation are associated with elevated inflammation markers, such as C-reactive protein (CRP), which correlates with depressive symptoms. In contrast, social interactions stimulate dopamine release, leading to reductions in depressive symptoms and improved life satisfaction by 30-40% (Pressman et al., 2005).

Strategies for Building Connection and Support in Recovery

Establishing strong social ties and cultivating new relationships can significantly improve mental health. Here are some practical strategies to integrate supportive connections into the recovery process.

Social Prescribing: A Formal Pathway to Connection

Social prescribing is now an evidence-based clinical pathway available through primary care in many countries, including Australia, the UK, and parts of North America. Rather than a medication, a GP or mental health clinician refers a patient to a "link worker" – a trained professional who co-designs a personalised plan connecting the individual to community-based activities proven to reduce depression and loneliness: arts groups, gardening programmes, volunteering, exercise classes, or walking groups.

A 2024 social identity framework published in Group Processes and Intergroup Relations (Haslam et al., 2024) explains why social prescribing works: it rebuilds a sense of group identity and personal purpose – two of the core psychological losses in depression – rather than simply providing social contact. The framework emphasises that social prescribing only succeeds when it cultivates a shared "social identity"; placing isolated individuals into group settings without authentic group belonging is ineffective. A 2025/2026 clinical trial ("Wellbeing While Waiting", 558 youth) found that social prescribing significantly improved behavioural difficulties and resilience over six months, but did not yield statistically significant reductions in primary anxiety or depressive symptoms compared to usual care. Social prescribing is therefore best understood as an adjunct that builds resilience and social connection, rather than a standalone treatment for depression.

How to access it: ask your GP, psychiatrist, or mental health team whether social prescribing is available in your area. In Australia, enquire about community health social workers; in the UK, ask about link worker referrals; in the US, community health centres and the Arts & Health field are expanding these services. If a formal programme is not available, the principles are the same: identify a community activity aligned with your values, attend regularly, and allow group membership to rebuild your sense of identity and belonging.

1. Group Therapy and Peer Support: Fostering Resilience Through Strengths and Solutions

Group therapy and peer support provide opportunities for shared learning, empathy, and encouragement. However, a balance is essential to avoid excessive focus on negative experiences. As Abigail Shrier wisely noted, "Thinking and talking about your problems all the time literally makes them grow". In group settings, it is crucial to build a solutions-oriented mindset that prevents rumination, which can amplify distress rather than alleviate it.

- Balanced sharing with a focus on growth: Group settings offer a platform to share struggles but also encourage members to explore pathways forward, focusing on strengths, solutions, and resilience. This approach nurtures resilience by helping individuals stay oriented toward positive actions.

- Perspective and positive reinforcement: Hearing others' stories and coping strategies provides perspective and reduces isolation, reinforcing a positive, supportive atmosphere. Celebrating small achievements within the group reinforces constructive thinking, reducing the risk of rumination.

- Creating a community of hope and empowerment: By focusing on victories, strengths, and strategies, group members build a shared sense of hope and resilience, supporting long-term mental health.

2. Strengthening Existing Relationships

Nurturing relationships with close friends and family members builds a dependable support network. High-quality relationships provide a safe space for honest communication, shared experiences, and emotional support, which are essential for strength.

- Regular check-ins: Scheduling weekly or bi-weekly conversations with friends or family members can reduce depressive symptoms by 20-30% (Thoits, 2011). These consistent interactions offer an opportunity to share challenges and receive encouragement.

- Building emotional intimacy: Building trust and vulnerability in relationships builds stronger bonds, reducing cortisol levels and boosting mood by 20-40%. A sense of safety within close relationships has significant positive effects on mental health (Pietromonaco et al., 2013).

3. Expanding Social Networks

Joining new social groups or participating in community activities introduces novelty and variety, creating a fulfilling sense of belonging. Expanding one's social network also provides opportunities to connect over shared interests and purposes.

- Interest-based groups: Engaging in activities or hobbies with like-minded individuals can reduce depressive symptoms by 10-20% by stimulating dopamine release and providing a sense of accomplishment (Cruwys et al., 2014).

- Volunteering and community involvement: Volunteering improves self-esteem and life satisfaction by creating meaningful social roles. Studies suggest that volunteering reduces depression by 30% and contributes to a greater sense of purpose (Jenkinson et al., 2013).

Avoiding Rumination: Cultivating Constructive Focus in Recovery

While reflection can support understanding, constant rumination – repetitively thinking about problems – often intensifies distress and leads to negative mental cycles. Research indicates that rumination increases cortisol and undermines emotional strength, particularly in individuals managing depression (Nolen-Hoeksema et al., 2008).

Practical techniques for reducing rumination include:

- Practising solution-focused thinking: Instead of fixating on problems, direct your focus toward actionable steps. If you find yourself repeatedly thinking about a particular issue, ask, "What can I do right now to support myself?" This approach encourages forward momentum and empowers constructive focus.

- Mindfulness techniques: Mindfulness practices, such as deep breathing and meditation, help interrupt cycles of repetitive thinking. Regular mindfulness strengthens the brain's capacity to stay present, reducing the tendency to dwell on negative thoughts (Segal et al., 2013).

- Engaging in physical activity or creative hobbies: Physical activity and creativity can help redirect attention from ruminative thoughts. Exercise and creative engagement stimulate the brain's reward systems, improving mood and strength (Craft & Perna, 2004).
- Setting time limits for reflection: Allocating a specific time daily to reflect on challenges, such as 10-15 minutes, allows for necessary processing while preventing extended rumination sessions. This structure promotes emotional health and mental clarity.

How Connection Amplifies Other Healing Layers

Social support strengthens the impact of other therapeutic and lifestyle changes by improving strength, emotional regulation, and mental well-being. Here's how the connection works synergistically with other layers:

- Improved emotional regulation: Sharing emotions with a trusted support system decreases emotional reactivity and creates a buffer against stress.
- Increased motivation and accountability: Social relationships foster accountability for self-care practices, like therapy attendance, exercise, and goal-setting, boosting adherence and motivation.
- Resilience to future challenges: Strong social bonds act as a safety net, offering resources and emotional support that help individuals manage life's setbacks with strength.

Key Takeaways

- Social support as a core element of strength: Strong social connections reduce the risk of depression and improve life satisfaction, acting as protective buffers against stress.

- Group and peer support for recovery: Structured and peer-led groups provide understanding and encouragement, reinforcing a growth-focused mindset.
- Balanced focus in relationships: Constructively focusing on solutions and strengths in relationships builds strength and mitigates rumination, supporting mental wellness.

References

Cohen, S. (2004). Social relationships and health. American Psychologist, 59(8), 676–684.

Craft, L. L., & Perna, F. M. (2004). The benefits of exercise for the clinically depressed. Primary Care Companion to the Journal of Clinical Psychiatry, 6(3), 104–111.

Cruwys, T., et al. (2014). Social group memberships protect against future depression, alleviate depression symptoms and prevent depression relapse. Social Science & Medicine, 98, 179–186.

Holt-Lunstad, J., et al. (2010). Social relationships and mortality risk: A meta-analytic review. PLoS Med, 7(7), e1000316.

Jenkinson, C. E., et al. (2013). Is volunteering a public health intervention? A systematic review and meta-analysis of the health and survival of volunteers. BMC Public Health, 13, 773.

Nolen-Hoeksema, S., et al. (2008). Rethinking rumination. Perspectives on Psychological Science, 3(5), 400–424.

Pietromonaco, P. R., et al. (2013). What can we learn about close relationships and health from daily process research? Social and Personality Psychology Compass, 7(4), 315–331.

Pressman, S. D., et al. (2005). Loneliness, social network size, and immune response to influenza vaccination in college freshmen. Health Psychology, 24(3), 297–306.

Haslam, S. A., Haslam, C., Cruwys, T., Sharman, L. S., Hayes, S., Walter, Z., & Jetten, J. (2024). Tackling loneliness together: A three-tier social identity framework for social prescribing. Group Processes and

Intergroup Relations, 27(5). https://doi.org/10.1177/13684302241242434

Santini, Z. I., et al. (2020). The association between social relationships and depression: A systematic review. Journal of Affective Disorders, 260, 653–662

CHAPTER 20

Environmental Design for Emotional Wellness

"The environment is not separate from ourselves; we are a part of it, and it is a part of us." – Carl Jung, Psychological Reflections

"We shape our buildings; thereafter, they shape us." – Winston Churchill, Speech to the House of Lords, 1943

The Impact of the Environment on Mental Health

Our environment plays a key role in shaping our emotional well-being and mental clarity. Research highlights how factors like natural light, air quality, noise levels, and organisation can reduce stress, improve mood, and improve cognitive function. Designing a supportive environment not only builds peace but also strengthens resilience, creating a foundation for mental wellness and recovery from depression (Ulrich, 1984; Kaplan & Kaplan, 1989). The focus here is on the powerful effects of an intentional, healing environment.

Here are some of the key environmental factors affecting mental health:

- Light exposure and circadian rhythms: Light exposure is vital for regulating circadian rhythms, which in turn influence mood, sleep, and cognitive function. Natural sunlight helps regulate serotonin and melatonin production, both critical for mental stability and restful sleep.

- Research insight: Exposure to natural light improves mood by up to 30% and has been shown to alleviate symptoms of non-seasonal depression as well as Seasonal Affective Disorder (SAD) (Cajochen et al., 2011; Young, 2007).

- Practical application: To align circadian rhythms and maximise daily sunlight exposure, ideally in the morning. Set up workspaces near windows, and during winter months, consider using a light therapy lamp to maintain healthy serotonin levels.

- Avoiding blue light for better sleep and mood regulation: Blue light from screens and artificial lighting can disrupt melatonin production, which is essential for sleep. Evening exposure to blue light delays melatonin release, disrupting sleep onset and quality and impacting mood and cognitive function.

- Research insight: Studies show that avoiding blue light in the two hours before bed improves sleep quality by up to 30% (Cajochen et al., 2011; Chang et al., 2015).

- Practical application: To support natural melatonin production and improve sleep quality, minimise screen time in the evening or wear blue light-blocking glasses. Set devices to "night mode" and use warm-toned lighting after sunset.

- The calming effects of nature and greenery: Nature exposure and indoor greenery reduce anxiety and improve focus. Natural settings and elements lower cortisol, engaging the parasympathetic nervous system and supporting relaxation and mental clarity.

- Research insight: Even brief exposure to nature can reduce cortisol levels by 15-30%, and indoor plants help improve air quality and support relaxation (Ulrich, 1984; Kaplan & Kaplan, 1989).

- Practical application: Introduce plants, natural materials, or nature-themed art in living spaces. Spending time outdoors, even in urban parks, improves mood and reduces stress.

- CO_2 and air quality – insights from James Nestor: Poor ventilation leads to higher indoor CO_2 levels, which James Nestor, in Breath, links to cognitive impairment and fatigue. Elevated CO_2 in modern buildings can reduce concentration and contribute to feelings of stress and mental fog.

- Research insight: Poor air quality is associated with increased inflammation, a risk factor for depression, while clean air supports cognitive performance and reduces depressive symptoms by 20-30% (Power et al., 2015; Gao et al., 2017).

- Practical application: Regularly ventilate rooms and open windows and use HEPA filters to reduce indoor pollutants. Incorporate air-purifying plants like snake plants and spider plants, which help remove airborne toxins and volatile organic compounds (VOCs) from indoor air.

- Noise reduction for focus and calm: Chronic noise pollution increases stress and impedes cognitive performance. Reducing background noise improves relaxation, focus, and emotional stability, making it easier to maintain mental clarity and reduce stress.

- Research insight: Chronic exposure to noise pollution elevates cortisol, while quieter spaces improve focus and resilience by 15-25% (Stansfeld & Matheson, 2003).

- Practical application: Use noise-cancelling headphones, soundproofing materials, or white noise machines. Calming nature sounds can also help mask disruptive noise and support a sense of calm.

- The psychology of colour and emotional impact: The colours in our environment influence our mood and cognitive performance. Cooler colours, such as blues and greens, have calming effects, while warmer colours, like yellows, stimulate energy and positivity.

- Research insight: Calming colours such as blue and green can reduce anxiety and improve focus by 10-15%, while warmer colours, when used sparingly, can lift mood (Kwallek et al., 1996).

- Practical application: Blue and green tones can be used in bedrooms or relaxation areas to foster tranquillity, while warmer accents can be added to workspaces to stimulate focus and motivation.

- Decluttering and minimalist living for mental clarity: Clutter creates cognitive overload, increasing stress and hindering relaxation. A minimalist environment, free of excess, promotes mental clarity, reduces anxiety, and builds a peaceful atmosphere.

- Research insight: Cluttered spaces are linked to elevated cortisol levels, while organised, minimalist areas improve focus and reduce anxiety, improving mental health by up to 20% (Roe et al., 2013).

- Practical application: Regularly clear out unnecessary items, especially in spaces where you relax or work. Keep essential and meaningful items visible to build a sense of calm and purpose.

Creating a Healing Environment: Room-by-Room Guide

- Bedroom: Optimise for rest with blackout curtains, cool colour tones, and a "no electronics" rule. Aromatherapy, like lavender essential oil, can support relaxation before bed.
- Living area: Add greenery and remove clutter to create a peaceful atmosphere. Include meaningful decor, such as family photos or art, to create a comforting environment.
- Workspace: If possible, place your desk near natural light. Use organisation tools to minimise distractions, and consider using noise-cancelling headphones or nature soundscapes to improve focus.
- Bathroom: Maintain a clean, minimalist setup with calming colours. Consider adding humidity-loving plants like ferns to purify the air and improve relaxation.

How Environmental Design Amplifies Other Healing Layers

- Improved sleep and circadian rhythm alignment: By optimising light exposure and reducing evening blue light, you improve sleep hygiene and align circadian rhythms, which stabilise mood and energy levels.
- Reduced stress and enhanced calm: A decluttered, natural environment promotes mindfulness and calm, supporting emotional resilience and stress management.
- Increased cognitive clarity and focus: Organised, intentional spaces reduce mental overload, making it easier to focus on therapeutic practices and lifestyle changes essential for depression recovery.

Key Takeaways

- Environment as a tool for wellness: A well-designed space reduces stress, improves mental clarity, and supports emotional stability.
- Light, nature, and air quality: Incorporating natural light, greenery, and purified air creates an environment that supports mental wellness.
- Mindful organisation: Decluttering, using calming colours, and managing noise contribute to a balanced, supportive space for mental recovery.

References

Bringslimark, T., Hartig, T., & Patil, G. G. (2009). The psychological benefits of indoor plants: A critical review of the experimental literature. Journal of Environmental Psychology, 29(4), 422–433.

Cajochen, C., Frey, S., Anders, D., Späti, J., Bues, M., Pross, A., ... & Stefani, O. (2011). Evening exposure to LED-backlit screens affects circadian physiology and sleep. Journal of Applied Physiology, 110(5), 1432–1438.

Gao, Y., Zhang, H., Luo, H., & Huang, H. (2017). Ambient air pollution exposures and depression: A review of epidemiological findings. Current Environmental Health Reports, 4(3), 213–226.

Kaplan, R., & Kaplan, S. (1989). The Experience of Nature: A psychological perspective. Cambridge University Press.

Kwallek, N., Lewis, C. M., & Robbins, A. S. (1996). Effects of office interior colour on workers' mood and productivity. Perceptual and Motor Skills, 83(2), 491–497.

Nestor, J. (2020). Breath: The new science of a lost art. Riverhead Books.

Power, M. C., Kioumourtzoglou, M. A., Hart, J. E., Okereke, O. I., Laden, F., & Weisskopf, M. G. (2015). The relation between air pollution and risk of cognitive decline: Results from the Nurses' Health Study. Environmental Health Perspectives, 123(3), 234–240.

Roe, J. J., Thompson, C. W., Aspinall, P. A., Brewer, M. J., Duff, E. I., Miller, D., & Clow, A. (2013). Green space and stress: Evidence from cortisol measures in deprived urban communities. International Journal of Environmental Research and Public Health, 10(9), 4086–4103.

Stansfeld, S. A., & Matheson, M. P. (2003). Noise pollution: Non-auditory effects on health. British Medical Bulletin, 68(1), 243–257.

Ulrich, R. S. (1984). View through a window may influence recovery from surgery. Science, 224(4647), 420–421.

CHAPTER 21

Progressive Relaxation Techniques for Emotional Stability

Introduction: The Importance of Relaxation in Mental Health

In depression recovery, managing stress and physical tension is important for building emotional strength and maintaining mental clarity. Progressive relaxation techniques, like Trauma Releasing Exercises (TRE) and progressive muscle relaxation (PMR), are powerful tools for reducing physical tension, increasing body awareness, and stabilising mood. By building a calm, balanced nervous system, these techniques support both mental and physical health, contributing to a combined, thorough approach to healing.

Understanding Progressive Relaxation and Its Benefits

- The mind-body connection in stress and depression: Depression is often linked to an overactive stress response, resulting in increased muscle tension, shallow breathing, and overall fatigue. Progressive relaxation techniques stimulate the parasympathetic nervous system (PNS), counteracting stress hormones like cortisol and reducing symptoms of anxiety and mood swings.

- Research insight: Studies indicate that activating the PNS through relaxation techniques can lower cortisol levels by 20-30%, easing depressive symptoms and emotional reactivity (Porges, 2009).

- Practical insight: Regular relaxation practice supports mental clarity, improves mood regulation, and helps transition the body to a restful, restorative state, aiding emotional well-being and strength.

- The role of the vagus nerve in relaxation: The vagus nerve is a vital component of the PNS and plays a central role in regulating relaxation and stress responses. Techniques that stimulate the vagus nerve, such as deep breathing, humming, and cold exposure, improve vagal tone, which is an indicator of strength and emotional stability.

- Research insight: High vagal tone is linked to a balanced stress response and improved heart rate variability (HRV), which can contribute to a 15-25% improvement in strength and emotional regulation (Porges, 2003).

- Practical application: Regularly practising exercises that stimulate the vagus nerve, such as diaphragmatic breathing, can build relaxation and strength over time.

Relaxation Techniques for Depression Recovery

- Progressive muscle relaxation (PMR): PMR involves tensing and then relaxing different muscle groups, supporting physical tension awareness and releasing stress stored in the body. PMR is effective for reducing anxiety and building deep relaxation.

- Research insight: PMR has been shown to decrease anxiety levels by 20-30% and improve relaxation by releasing muscle tension related to stress (Bernstein & Borkovec, 1973).

- Practical application: Start by focusing on the feet, gradually tensing and relaxing each muscle group as you move up the body. Practising PMR before bed can improve sleep quality and release daily stress.

- Trauma releasing exercises (TRE): TRE aims to release stress and tension stored in the body, particularly in cases of trauma. It uses exercises that encourage controlled shaking or tremoring, releasing tension and building relaxation.

- Research insight: Studies indicate that TRE can reduce stress symptoms and improve emotional regulation by up to 40%, releasing physical tension from trauma (Berceli & Napoli, 2006).

- Practical application: Practicing TRE two to three times a week can help reduce chronic stress and support calm, especially for those with trauma-related muscle tension.

- Diaphragmatic (deep) breathing: Deep breathing stimulates the vagus nerve, activating the PNS and shifting the body out of a stress response. Focusing on slow, controlled breaths from the diaphragm increases oxygen flow, lowers heart rate, and calms the mind.

- Research insight: Diaphragmatic breathing has been shown to improve HRV and reduce stress by 20-40%, improving mood stability and decreasing depressive symptoms (Jerath et al., 2006).

- Practical application: Practice deep breathing by inhaling through the nose for a count of four, holding for two, and exhaling through the mouth for a count of six. Aim for 5-10 minutes daily, especially during stressful moments.

- Neuroacoustic Sound Therapy: Neuroacoustic therapy uses sound frequencies to guide the brain into relaxed states. Promoting brainwave activity associated with calm and focus can reduce stress, improve sleep quality, and support mood stability.

- Research insight: Neuroacoustic therapy has been linked to 20-30% improvements in relaxation and sleep quality (Leeds, 2010).

- Practical application: To support relaxation and better sleep, use a sound therapy app or playlist with calming frequencies during meditation or bedtime.

- Aromatherapy and essential oils: Aromatherapy, particularly with essential oils like lavender, helps induce relaxation by interacting with the brain's limbic system, governing mood and emotions. Some essential oils, such as lavender, can cross the blood-brain barrier, exerting calming effects on the mind and body.

- Research insight: Inhaling lavender essential oil has been shown to reduce anxiety and improve sleep quality by 15-25% (Koulivand et al., 2013).

- Practical application: Use a diffuser with calming essential oils in your relaxation space, or place a few drops on a cotton ball nearby during meditation or bedtime.

- Magnesium as a muscle relaxant: Magnesium is a mineral known for its muscle-relaxing properties. It plays a vital role in reducing tension and aiding recovery from stress. Magnesium deficiency has been linked to increased stress responses, while supplementation has been shown to reduce muscle cramps, tension, and headaches, supporting overall relaxation.

- Research insight: Supplementing with magnesium has been found to improve relaxation by reducing muscle tension and stress by 10-15% (Barbagallo & Dominguez, 2010).

- Practical application: Incorporate magnesium-rich foods, such as leafy greens and nuts, into your diet, or consider magnesium supplements as recommended by a healthcare provider for added relaxation support.

Incorporating Relaxation Techniques into Daily Life

- Set a relaxation routine: Incorporate one or more relaxation techniques into your daily routine, such as starting the day with deep breathing or ending it with PMR.
- Use reminders for consistency: Set phone reminders for relaxation breaks to create a habit of calmness and strength.
- Adapt techniques to situational needs: Use quick techniques like deep breathing for immediate stress relief while reserving longer practices like PMR or TRE for relaxation in the evening.

How Relaxation Techniques Amplify Other Healing Layers

- Enhanced emotional regulation: Relaxation techniques release stored physical tension, supporting emotional stability and reinforcing practices like mindfulness and cognitive behavioural therapy (CBT).
- Improved sleep quality and recovery: Practising relaxation before bed supports restful sleep, which is essential for mood stability and cognitive clarity.
- Reduced physical symptoms of depression: Many people with depression experience physical symptoms, such as muscle pain and fatigue. Relaxation techniques ease muscular tension, providing whole-person support for recovery.

Key Takeaways

- The power of relaxation in depression recovery: Regular relaxation techniques help reduce physical tension, improve emotional regulation, and decrease stress responses.

- Practical techniques for daily life: Techniques like PMR, TRE, deep breathing, neuroacoustic therapy, and magnesium supplementation offer accessible ways to integrate relaxation into daily routines.
- Building strength through consistency: Consistent relaxation practice builds strength, supports sleep quality, and promotes mental and physical wellness.

References

Barbagallo, M., & Dominguez, L. J. (2010). Magnesium and aging. Current Pharmaceutical Design, 16(7), 832–839.

Berceli, D., & Napoli, M. (2006). A proposal for a mindful-based trauma prevention programme for social work professionals. Journal of Trauma Practice, 5(1), 25–40.

Bernstein, D. A., & Borkovec, T. D. (1973). Progressive relaxation training: A manual for the helping professions. Champaign, IL: Research Press.

Jerath, R., et al. (2006). Physiology of long pranayamic breathing: Neural respiratory elements may provide a mechanism that explains how slow breathing shifts the autonomic nervous system. Medical Hypotheses, 67(3), 566–571.

Koulivand, P. H., et al. (2013). Lavender and the nervous system. Evidence-Based Complementary and Alternative Medicine, 2013.

Leeds, J. (2010). The Power of Sound: How to manage your personal soundscape for a vital, productive, and healthy life. Healing Arts Press.

Porges, S. W. (2003). The polyvagal theory: Phylogenetic contributions to social behavior. Physiology & Behavior, 79(3), 503–513.

CHAPTER 22

How Pets Support Depression Recovery

Introduction: Pets as Companions in Depression Recovery

Pets bring more than just companionship – they provide a sense of purpose, comfort, and emotional support, all of which are important for depression recovery. For those experiencing depressive symptoms, pets can alleviate loneliness, promote physical activity, and establish a comforting routine. Pets' non-judgemental presence and consistent companionship offer a safe space to process emotions. Here, we examine the science behind pet therapy and details how pets contribute to emotional stability, social connection, and physical health, making them valuable allies in combined depression recovery.

The Science of Animal Companionship and Depression Relief

1. Alleviating Depression Symptoms through Pet Interaction

Pet interaction provides more than a temporary mood boost – it supports essential emotional regulation. Research shows that engaging with pets can reduce cortisol, the primary stress hormone, while boosting oxytocin, serotonin, and dopamine – neurotransmitters associated with feelings of happiness, calm, and stability.

Studies indicate that pet ownership is linked to a 50% reduction in depressive episodes. Oxytocin, known as the "bonding hormone", naturally calms the nervous system, creating a buffer against symptoms of sadness and isolation (Friedmann & Son, 2009; Wood et al., 2015).

Pets offer unconditional companionship that can improve self-esteem for individuals who struggle with self-worth. Daily interactions with pets can also interrupt negative thought loops and help reduce rumination, a common challenge in depression.

2. Countering Isolation and Social Withdrawal

Depression often leads to social isolation, but pets act as a bridge to the outside world, providing low-pressure opportunities to connect with others. Dog owners usually meet people at parks or pet events, which helps reduce loneliness and create a sense of community.

Studies show that pet ownership can reduce feelings of isolation by up to 50%, which positively impacts mental health and strength (McNicholas & Collis, 2006).

Simple social interactions fostered by pet ownership, even short exchanges with other pet owners, provide connection without the intensity or expectations that may feel overwhelming for those with depression.

3. Physical Health Benefits and Their Impact on Mood

Pets, particularly dogs, encourage physical activity through daily walks. These walks provide the dual benefits of exercise and outdoor exposure, both of which are known mood stabilisers. Movement releases endorphins, the body's natural mood enhancers, while sunlight supports circadian rhythm regulation, which is important for maintaining energy and mental clarity.

Regular dog walkers report 20-30% improvements in mood and physical health, with added benefits for circadian rhythms that improve sleep and overall mental clarity (Cutt et al., 2008; Ranganathan et al., 2015).

Developing a daily routine with a pet adds structure and purpose, which can improve motivation and stability. For those with depression, establishing consistent, small achievements through pet care can help restore confidence and combat feelings of helplessness.

Types of Therapeutic Pets and Their Unique Benefits for Depression Recovery

1. Emotional Support Animals (ESAs)

Emotional Support Animals offer companionship and comfort for those with mental health conditions. Though not trained for specific tasks, their presence can significantly reduce anxiety and support calm. Interacting with ESAs can lower depression and anxiety symptoms by up to 40%, providing crucial support on difficult days (Wells, 2009). Registering an ESA allows individuals to bring pets into restricted settings, such as housing or travel situations, so their support is accessible in varied environments.

2. Therapy Animals for Structured Support

Therapy animals are trained to provide comfort in settings such as hospitals, nursing homes, schools, and therapy sessions. In depression recovery, therapy animals can reduce stress and encourage social engagement, helping individuals feel more relaxed and less isolated.

In clinical settings, therapy animals reduce stress and anxiety by 25-35% (Barker et al., 2003), aiding emotional stability and encouraging participation in group settings. Participating in programmes with therapy animals or community animal therapy events can build social skills, ease anxiety, and build a sense of support, encouraging more active engagement in social and therapeutic activities.

3. Service Animals for Complex Depression Support

Service animals provide specialised support for severe mental health needs, such as managing symptoms of PTSD or severe anxiety. These animals are trained to perform tasks that support emotional stability, such as providing tactile comfort or interrupting panic attacks, making them highly beneficial for individuals with treatment-resistant depression or complex depressive symptoms.

Service animals for mental health reduce stress and anxiety by up to 60% for conditions like PTSD (Yount et al., 2012; Rodriguez et al., 2019). For those with severe depression, service animals offer life-changing assistance by making daily activities more manageable and reducing the risk of depressive episodes.

Integrating Pets into Depression Recovery Routines

- Low-pressure interaction: For days when energy or motivation is low, passive interactions, like lying beside a pet or watching them play, provide grounding and relaxation without requiring intense effort.

- Mindful pet interaction: Use pet care as a mindfulness practice. Spend a few minutes petting or observing your pet, focusing on the sensory details such as their fur or breathing. This present-focused exercise supports calm and reduces stress.

- Outdoor activities for mood boost: Engage in regular outdoor activities, like dog walks or park trips. Exposure to natural light and fresh air helps regulate circadian rhythms and improves energy levels, both of which are beneficial for mood.

Special Considerations for Pet Ownership with Depression

- Managing pet responsibilities during relapses: Depression can affect the ability to care for pets, particularly during relapses consistently. For those concerned about this, seeking support from friends or family for pet care during difficult periods can reduce stress. Additionally, planning for a more straightforward care routine during challenging times can help avoid feeling overwhelmed.
- Considering alternatives for those unable to own pets: For individuals who cannot own a pet, virtual pet therapy sessions or community-based programmes offer similar benefits without the full-time commitment. Facilities that offer pet interaction or animal-assisted therapy are excellent alternatives for experiencing the joy and comfort of animal companionship.

Enhancing Depression Recovery with Pet Therapy in Layered Healing

- Emotional regulation and therapy synergy: Pets can serve as therapeutic partners, especially in settings like Cognitive Behavioural Therapy (CBT). Their comforting presence can reduce therapy-related anxiety, creating a supportive, judgement-free space for processing emotions.

- Routine stability and motivation: Pet care responsibility builds a consistent routine and encourages motivation to maintain other mental health strategies, such as exercise and sleep hygiene.
- Physical health benefits: Regular physical activity and sunlight exposure, such as walking or playing with pets, boost cognitive function and mood, creating foundational support for mental wellness.

Key Takeaways

- Pets as companions in depression recovery: Pets offer unconditional companionship that alleviates feelings of loneliness, low self-esteem, and isolation, making them uniquely suited for depression recovery.
- Multi-combined benefits: From ESAs to service animals, pets provide specific support for those with depression, improving emotional stability, motivation, and strength.
- Practical routine integration: Structured routines and mindful interaction with pets support calm, self-awareness, and consistency, aligning well with combined healing approaches for managing depression.

References

Barker, S. B., et al. (2003). Therapeutic aspects of human-companion animal interactions. Psychiatric Times, 20(3), 28–36.

Beetz, A., et al. (2012). Psychosocial and psychophysiological effects of human-animal interactions: The possible role of oxytocin. Frontiers in Psychology, 3, 234.

Cutt, H., et al. (2008). Dog ownership, health, and physical activity: A critical review of the literature. Health & Place, 14(1), 1–15.

McNicholas, J., & Collis, G. M. (2006). Animals as social supports: Insights for mobilising and nurturing social support in relationships with companion animals. Society and Animals, 14(4), 385–404.

Rodriguez, K. E., et al. (2019). The effect of service dogs on PTSD symptomology in military veterans. Psychiatry Research, 274, 157–164.

CHAPTER 23

Creating a Personalised Healing Plan

Introduction: Why Personalisation and Layering Matter in Depression Recovery

Every person's process to mental health recovery is unique and shaped by individual needs, lifestyle, and circumstances. A personalised healing plan allows you to prioritise and integrate therapeutic layers from earlier chapters – like sleep, nutrition, movement, sunlight, and nature exposure – ensuring that each one maximises its impact. This approach emphasises layering, or combining supportive therapies, to create a cumulative effect that strengthens the plan and makes it sustainable. Research shows that integrating multiple therapeutic approaches can lead to a 40-60% greater improvement in mental health than using single methods alone (Smith et al., 2021). This chapter will guide you through creating a layered healing plan that incorporates core therapies alongside psychotherapy, tailored to your needs and goals for a balanced, adaptable approach to recovery.

The Benefits of a Personalised and Layered Approach to Healing

Personalising a healing plan and layering therapeutic elements offer numerous scientifically supported benefits:

- Enhanced motivation and engagement: Therapy aligned with individual needs and goals naturally builds engagement. Layering foundational therapies – such as exercise, sleep, and nutrition – creates a cumulative effect, where improvements in one area reinforce motivation and adherence to others. Studies suggest that tailored therapies can increase adherence by 25-40% (Jones et al., 2018).
- Addressing multiple symptoms simultaneously: Layering allows you to target multiple areas of well-being, such as mood, energy, and physical health, at once. Better sleep, for example, can lead to improved mood and energy, reinforcing the effectiveness of additional layers.
- Sustainable, incremental progress: Smaller, layered steps in each area are easier to sustain over time. Layering enables you to build on each success, with research showing that incremental progress boosts long-term adherence by up to 30% (Geller et al., 2021).

This layered approach amplifies the benefits of each therapy, providing a flexible, sustainable path to healing that can adapt as your needs evolve.

Steps for Developing Your Personalised, Layered Healing Plan

Step 1: Assess Your Current Needs and Goals

As suggested in Chapter 1, an assessment of your current state clarifies where personalisation and layering would be most beneficial.

- Using assessments: Baseline tools like the Depression Anxiety Stress Scale (DASS21), mood journals, or health evaluations highlight areas for improvement and indicate where layering might offer the most benefit. For instance, if sleep and stress are primary concerns, a layered approach might include sleep optimisation combined with mindfulness practices.

- Setting goals: Define specific, measurable goals, like "increasing daily exposure to natural light" or "improving sleep quality by 30%". Setting benchmarks creates a focused direction for layering and provides a structured way to track progress.

Step 2: Identify Core Layers for Your Recovery

Drawing from earlier chapters, select the core layers most relevant to your well-being. Each chapter has introduced essential therapeutic layers that can be prioritised and adapted to meet your needs:

- Sleep optimisation as a foundation (Chapter 4): Improved sleep quality reduces depressive symptoms and improves other layers, such as mood and energy, making it an ideal foundation. Techniques like consistent bedtime routines or melatonin support may be particularly effective if sleep disruption is a core issue. Studies show that sleep quality improvements can reduce depressive symptoms by 20-50% (Irwin, 2015).

- Movement and Exercise (Chapter 5): Physical activity significantly alleviates depressive symptoms, with improvements of up to 50% (Schuch et al., 2018). For those with low energy or mood, prioritising movement strengthens other therapeutic areas, such as nutritional goals and strength.

- Nutrition and blood sugar stability (Chapters 6 and 7): A stable, nutrient-rich diet is essential for balanced mood and energy. Nutritional improvements, like increasing omega-3s or anti-inflammatory foods, are linked to mood improvements of up to 35% (Firth et al., 2020). Combining these dietary adjustments with exercise and sleep hygiene strengthens overall stability and well-being.

- Sunlight and time in nature (Chapter 8): Exposure to natural light and time spent in nature are associated with improved mood, reduced stress, and better mental clarity. Natural light exposure helps regulate circadian rhythms, aiding sleep quality and supporting emotional resilience. Spending time in nature, even just 20 minutes a day, has been shown to lower cortisol levels, reducing anxiety and depressive symptoms by 20-30% (Ulrich et al., 1991). When combined with exercise or mindfulness, sunlight and nature provide a strong foundation for mental wellness.

By selecting core layers that address high-impact areas, you maximise the overall benefits of your healing plan.

Step 3: Integrate Psychotherapy as a Key Layer in Your Plan

Alongside physical wellness layers, psychotherapy provides essential support for addressing underlying emotional and cognitive patterns that contribute to depression. Psychotherapy works synergistically with other therapeutic elements by increasing emotional strength, offering coping strategies, and building lasting mental health improvements.

- Somatic and bottom-up therapies: Somatic therapies, such as somatic experiencing or trauma-release exercises (TRE), focus on the body's response to emotional distress, allowing stress to release from the body. When layered with movement and grounding techniques, these therapies help process trauma, reduce depressive symptoms, and improve mood stability.

- Relational and emotional processing therapies: Approaches such as Gestalt or dynamic therapy enhance emotional awareness and relational resilience, making it easier to engage in lifestyle adjustments like diet or exercise routines. Studies indicate that those who combine talk therapy with physical wellness practices report longer-lasting improvements and higher adherence to treatment (Cuijpers et al., 2019).

Psychotherapy complements other layers, creating an emotionally stable and supportive foundation for sustained healing.

Step 4: Customise Each Layer for Your Lifestyle

Once you've chosen core layers, adapt each to fit your unique schedule, preferences, and resources. This layering approach also allows you to see how one adjustment can positively affect another, reinforcing each layer's effect.

- Adapting exercise: If time is limited, even a 10-minute high-intensity session can provide a 25% boost in mood and energy (Mammen & Faulkner, 2013). These shorter sessions are often easier to combine with mindfulness techniques, like focusing on breathing during stretching.

- Creating a sleep routine: Establishing a sleep routine that includes relaxing activities like reading or gentle stretching has been shown to improve sleep quality by 15-30% (Irwin, 2015). A calming pre-sleep routine supports both sleep quality and daily energy.

- Choosing nutritional goals: Small dietary adjustments, such as adding an anti-inflammatory meal per day, can impact mood by up to 35% (Firth et al., 2020). When combined with exercise or mindfulness, dietary improvements amplify overall well-being.

Customising each layer ensures that your healing plan remains adaptable, flexible, and easy to sustain.

Step 5: Track Progress and Make Adjustments as Needed

Tracking progress, as suggested in Chapter 3, allows you to monitor each layer's contribution to overall health and identify areas that may need adjustment. For instance, improved sleep can enhance mood, making it easier to engage in other layers like movement and nutrition.

- Setting up weekly check-ins: Reflecting weekly on questions like "What went well?" and "What adjustments are needed?" can increase adherence by up to 25% (Thompson et al., 2020). This reinforces the cumulative benefits of layering by allowing you to adapt as needed.
- Using technology for tracking: Apps for tracking sleep or physical activity offer data-driven insights, helping you identify patterns and adjust layers for optimal results.

Regular tracking ensures that your healing plan is responsive to your needs, making it an effective long-term strategy.

Step 6: Build a Support System That Reinforces Layered Healing

Supportive relationships provide stability and motivation. As highlighted in Chapter 19, social support is invaluable to recovery, helping to reduce the risk of relapse and improve overall health. Research shows that social support can reduce the likelihood of relapse by up to 50% (Lakey & Orehek, 2011).

- Sharing goals with trusted support: Sharing your combined goals with friends or family increases accountability, reduces isolation, and helps sustain your plan through challenges.

- Community resources and professional guidance: Support groups, wellness workshops, or professional guidance introduce new perspectives that reinforce your healing process. Professional support, in particular, provides expertise in refining and adjusting therapeutic layers as your needs evolve.

Supportive relationships bolster resilience and improve the sustainability of your combined healing plan.

Practical Example of a Layered, Personalised Healing Plan

In this example, the core goal is to improve emotional stability, strength, and engagement. Based on a personal assessment of high-impact needs, the following healing layers were selected to work together: psychotherapy, sleep, movement, nutrition, sunlight, and mindfulness. The personalised actions below explain how each layer is applied in practice.

- Personalised actions:
- Psychotherapy: Attend weekly sessions in somatic or trauma-release therapy to address underlying stress and emotional strength.
- Sleep: Follow a consistent bedtime routine with a meditation app, aiming to improve sleep quality by 30%.
- Nutrition: Incorporate nutrient-dense foods, such as leafy greens and omega-3s, to boost mood by 25-35%.
- Movement: A daily 15-minute walk and weekly yoga are linked to mood enhancement by 20-50%.
- Sunlight and nature: Spend at least 20 minutes each day outdoors, exposed to natural light and nature, aiming to

improve mood by 20-30%.

- Mindfulness: Daily gratitude journaling can reduce depressive symptoms by 15-20% (Emmons & McCullough, 2003).
- Tracking: Use a journal to record weekly mood, energy, and sleep quality.
- Support: Join a monthly support group and schedule bi-weekly check-ins with a close friend.

This structured yet flexible plan aligns each layer with specific goals, creating a clear path to enhanced mood and energy.

How Layering Amplifies Other Healing Layers

Maximising Impact: Prioritising high-impact areas like sunlight and nature, combined with exercise and psychotherapy, reinforces cumulative benefits across all layers.

Enhancing Motivation and Consistency: Layered approaches increase engagement, with studies showing 25-50% higher adherence (Geller et al., 2021).

Providing Flexibility and Adaptability: Regular tracking and layering prevent burnout, creating a balanced, sustainable approach to healing.

Key Takeaways

- Personalisation and layering increase engagement: A customised, combined plan is easier to maintain and strengthens the effect of each therapeutic element.
- Flexibility and adaptability build long-term success: Adjusting each layer ensures sustainable progress.

- Support and accountability are essential: Building a support network reinforces resilience, reducing the risk of relapse.

Next Steps

- Set initial goals: Define your immediate and long-term recovery objectives.
- Choose core layers: Identify high-impact layers from earlier chapters to support your goals.
- Build your support system: Engage trusted friends, family, or professionals to foster accountability.

By layering and personalising each aspect of your healing plan, you create a pathway that is adaptable to your life, goals, and strengths. This makes recovery achievable, flexible, and sustainable.

References

Emmons, R. A., & McCullough, M. E. (2003). Counting blessings versus burdens: An experimental investigation of gratitude and subjective well-being in daily life. Journal of Personality and Social Psychology, 84(2), 377–389.

Firth, J., Gangwisch, J. E., Borsini, A., Wootton, R. E., & Mayer, E. A. (2020). Food and mood: How diet and nutrition affect mental health? BMJ, 369, m2382.

Geller, A., Strauss, M., & Goodman, L. (2021). Long-term outcomes of individualized interventions for mood disorders. Psychological Science, 12(4), 229–247.

Goyal, M., Singh, S., Sibinga, E. M., et al. (2014). Meditation programs for psychological stress and health: A systematic review and meta-analysis. JAMA Internal Medicine, 174(3), 357–368.

Irwin, M. R. (2015). Why sleep is important for health: A psychoneuroimmunology perspective. Annual Review of Psychology,

66, 143–172.

Jones, D. R., & Sinclair, R. (2018). Engaging clients through personalized approaches in therapy. Journal of Clinical Psychology, 10(2), 184–200.

Lakey, B., & Orehek, E. (2011). Relational regulation theory: A new approach to explain the link between perceived social support and mental health. Psychological Review, 118(3), 482–495.

Mammen, G., & Faulkner, G. (2013). Physical activity and the prevention of depression: A systematic review of prospective studies. American Journal of Preventive Medicine, 45(5), 649–657.

Schuch, F. B., Vancampfort, D., Firth, J., Rosenbaum, S., Ward, P. B., Silva, E. S., & Stubbs, B. (2018). Physical activity and incident depression: A meta-analysis of prospective cohort studies. American Journal of Psychiatry, 175(7), 631–648.

Smith, J. K., Adams, J., & Thompson, A. (2021). Combined therapeutic approaches in mental health treatment: A meta-analysis. Journal of Integrative Mental Health, 5(3), 241–256.

Thompson, A., Rosenberg, H., & Sheridan, M. (2020). The effectiveness of self-monitoring in adherence to personalized therapeutic plans. Journal of Behavioral Health, 4(2), 87–94.

Ulrich, R. S., Simons, R. F., Losito, B. D., Fiorito, E., Miles, M. A., & Zelson, M. (1991). Stress recovery during exposure to natural and urban environments. Journal of Environmental Psychology, 11(3), 201–230.

CHAPTER 24

Understanding Relapse and Building a Safety Net

Introduction: Why Relapse Prevention is Crucial

Relapse is a common concern in depression recovery, with studies indicating that up to 60% of individuals may experience recurrence within two years after initial improvement (Hardeveld et al., 2010). However, proactive relapse prevention strategies can reduce this risk, supporting sustained recovery and strength. A relapse prevention plan involves creating a personal safety net, tracking early warning signs, and building coping mechanisms – including a focus on diet, exercise, and sleep – to maintain stability. This chapter provides guidance on crafting a comprehensive relapse prevention plan to help you respond to challenges with confidence and flexibility.

Understanding Relapse in Depression Recovery

Relapse is the recurrence of depressive symptoms after a period of improvement. For those on a recovery process, relapse can feel discouraging, but it's essential to view it as part of the process, not a failure. Structured prevention methods can reduce relapse rates by 30-50% (Clarke et al., 2015). Factors that commonly contribute to relapse include:

- Stressful life events: High-stress events, such as relationship changes, work pressures, or significant life transitions, can increase relapse risk by up to 40%, particularly when coping mechanisms are limited (Monroe & Harkness, 2011).
- Changes in routine: Disruptions to stabilising routines, like sleep, exercise, or social habits, can trigger symptoms. For many, routine offers structure that helps stabilise mood and behaviour.
- Physical health factors: Poor diet, inconsistent exercise, and lack of quality sleep are all linked to increased relapse rates. Physical and mental health are closely connected, and habits like good nutrition, regular movement, and sleep hygiene influence mood stability.

Understanding these triggers enables you to build a proactive approach that prioritises preventive care, particularly in the areas of physical health and emotional resilience.

Steps to Build Your Relapse Prevention Plan

Step 1: Identify Early Warning Signs

Recognising early warning signs, which often appear as subtle changes in mood, thought patterns, or behaviours, can prevent symptoms from escalating.

- Common warning signs: Warning signs may include increased irritability, fatigue, and a return of negative thinking patterns – often appearing weeks before a full relapse (Judd et al., 2000). Additionally, reduced interest in daily routines, sleep disturbances, and changes in appetite can also be indicators.

- Tracking symptoms: Regular tracking, whether through a mood-tracking app, journal, or self-assessment tool, helps detect patterns. Studies show that daily tracking improves self-awareness and intervention efficacy by up to 25% (Wichers et al., 2011).

- Practising self-reflection – set aside time each day or week to reflect on your mood, physical energy, and behaviours: These reflections can reveal patterns, making it easier to adjust your plan as needed, such as by increasing self-care or engaging with your support network.

Identifying early signs enables timely intervention, reducing the likelihood of a full relapse.

Step 2: Create a Safety Net of Supportive Practices

A well-rounded safety net includes diet, exercise, and sleep, as well as social support and mindfulness practices. These foundational practices provide resilience in times of vulnerability and support stable mental health.

- Mindfulness and relaxation: Practicing mindfulness meditation, deep breathing, or progressive muscle relaxation can reduce relapse rates by up to 50% by helping you manage stress more effectively (Segal et al., 2010). Integrating mindfulness into your daily routine supports emotional stability and strength.

- Good nutrition: A balanced, anti-inflammatory diet, rich in whole foods, protein, and essential nutrients like omega-3 fatty acids, can improve mood stability. Research links a well-rounded diet to a 30% reduction in depressive symptoms (Firth et al., 2020). Regular, nourishing meals can help maintain energy levels and stabilise blood sugar, which in turn supports mental clarity and emotional balance.

- Regular physical activity: Exercise has been shown to decrease depressive symptoms by 20-40% and can act as a protective factor against relapse (Schuch et al., 2018). Even moderate activity, like a daily walk, cycling, or yoga, provides mood-boosting benefits, increases energy, and helps reduce stress.

- Sleep hygiene: Quality sleep is important for emotional stability and mental health, as it allows the brain to process emotions and repair itself. Sleep hygiene, such as maintaining a consistent bedtime and avoiding screens before sleep, supports deep, restorative sleep. Research shows that improved sleep quality can reduce depressive symptoms by 20-50% (Irwin, 2015).

- Social connections: Engaging with a support network lowers relapse risk by up to 30%, as social interaction mitigates isolation and provides accountability (Lakey & Orehek, 2011). Regular check-ins with friends, family, or support groups offer encouragement and reinforce strength.

These supportive practices create a foundation that helps maintain recovery even during periods of increased stress or challenge.

Step 3: Develop a Crisis Plan for High-Risk Situations

A crisis plan is essential for handling periods of acute distress. This plan includes steps and contacts you can rely on to navigate challenging times with clarity and support.

- Identifying high-risk situations: Recognise events or situations that may increase vulnerability, such as anniversaries of traumatic events, significant life changes, or times of high stress. Being prepared for these situations reduces their emotional impact and helps you maintain stability.

- Crisis response steps: Outline a series of steps to take during high-stress moments, such as grounding exercises, reaching out to a friend, or using a relaxation app. Studies show that having a crisis plan reduces symptom escalation by 25-35% during challenging periods (Stanley et al., 2008).

- Emergency contacts: List essential contacts, including mental health professionals, crisis hotlines, and trusted friends or family members. Knowing who to reach out to during a crisis can help prevent isolation and helps timely intervention.

A crisis plan provides a structured approach to handling difficult situations. It helps you maintain composure and minimise the impact of high-stress moments.

Step 4: Regularly Review and Adjust Your Plan

Relapse prevention plans need to be dynamic, adjusting as your needs evolve. Regular review ensures that your plan remains practical and relevant.

- Monthly self-assessments: Use self-assessment tools like the DASS21 monthly to track changes in mental health and identify areas that need adjustment. Consistent self-assessment reduces relapse risk by 20% (Lovibond & Lovibond, 1995) and helps you recognise subtle shifts in health.

- Adapting to life changes: Your life circumstances and stressors will change over time. Adjust your plan as needed to incorporate new coping skills or address current challenges.

- Celebrating progress: Recognising achievements, even small ones, reinforces progress and builds confidence. Celebrating milestones strengthens commitment to recovery and enhances motivation and strength.

By consistently reviewing your plan, you can ensure that it remains responsive to your current needs and supportive of your long-term mental health.

Practical Example of a Relapse Prevention Plan

Here's an example of a structured relapse prevention plan that integrates diet, exercise, sleep, supportive practices, and crisis management. When you notice certain warning signs, such as an increase in negative thinking, sleep disturbances, and irritability, these are some supportive practices you can turn to:

- Diet: Maintain a balanced diet with regular, nutrient-dense meals, such as incorporating omega-3-rich foods like salmon or walnuts.
- Exercise: Engage in moderate activity, like a daily 15-minute walk, and aim for weekly yoga sessions to sustain energy and support mood.
- Sleep: Establish a calming pre-sleep routine, like reading or meditating, aiming for seven to eight hours of restful sleep.
- Mindfulness: Practice mindfulness exercises, like 10 minutes of deep breathing, three times a week.
- Social support: Schedule bi-weekly check-ins with a trusted friend or family member.

Here is an example crisis plan you can implement:

- Step 1: Engage in grounding exercises (e.g., deep breathing for five minutes).
- Step 2: Call a trusted friend or crisis hotline.
- Step 3: Use a mental health app with relaxation exercises or guided meditation.

It is important to conduct regular reviews of your health. Track your mood and energy levels daily with a journal or app and complete the DASS21 monthly for ongoing self-assessment.

This example provides clear steps and resources, offering a safety net that supports strength against potential relapse triggers.

How Relapse Prevention Amplifies Other Healing Layers

A relapse prevention plan not only supports recovery but strengthens other foundational layers in your healing plan, creating a thorough approach to wellness:

- Enhancing physical health: By prioritising diet, exercise, and sleep, you can reinforce mental health stability and strength and reduce the risk of relapse.

- Improving emotional awareness: Recognising warning signs and tracking mood increases emotional awareness, enables earlier intervention, and helps sustain mood stability.

- Building strength: A structured safety net of supportive practices helps you respond constructively to life's challenges, reinforcing your overall approach to recovery.

- Fostering long-term engagement: Regular self-assessment and adaptation build a proactive, engaged approach, improving motivation to maintain recovery over time.

Key Takeaways

- Recognising warning signs is important: Early identification of warning signs enables prompt action, preventing symptoms from escalating into a full relapse.

- Good diet, exercise, and sleep are foundational: Physical health directly impacts mental health, and balanced nutrition, regular activity, and quality sleep reinforce stability.

- A crisis plan provides stability: Defining steps for high-risk situations ensures you are equipped to manage stress effectively.
- Consistent review strengthens recovery: Regular self-assessment and adaptation keep your plan responsive to changing needs.

Next Steps

- Identify personal triggers: Reflect on past experiences to identify potential relapse triggers unique to your situation.
- Build a crisis plan: Outline key steps and contacts to rely on during high-stress situations.
- Establish regular check-ins: Use mood tracking, dietary monitoring, and monthly assessments to monitor progress and adjust as needed.

A well-rounded relapse prevention plan, with attention to diet, exercise, and sleep, provides a strong safety net that helps you to handle challenges confidently and maintain recovery over the long term. This proactive approach ensures that even if setbacks occur, you're equipped with the tools and support needed to continue moving forward.

References

Clarke, G., Hornbrook, M., Lynch, F., Polen, M., Gale, J., O'Connor, E., & Seeley, J. (2015). A randomized effectiveness trial of brief cognitive-behavioral therapy for depressed adolescents receiving antidepressant medication. Journal of the American Academy of Child

& Adolescent Psychiatry, 54(11), 1020–1029.

Firth, J., Gangwisch, J. E., Borsini, A., Wootton, R. E., & Mayer, E. A. (2020). Food and mood: How diet and nutrition affect mental wellbeing? BMJ, 369, m2382.

Hardeveld, F., Spijker, J., De Graaf, R., Nolen, W. A., & Beekman, A. T. F. (2010). Recurrence of major depressive disorder and its predictors in the general population: Results from the Netherlands Mental Health Survey and Incidence Study (NEMESIS). Psychological Medicine, 40(2), 211–219.

Irwin, M. R. (2015). Why sleep is important for health: A psychoneuroimmunology perspective. Annual Review of Psychology, 66, 143–172.

Judd, L. L., Akiskal, H. S., & Schettler, P. J. (2000). Psychosocial disability during the long-term course of unipolar major depressive disorder. Archives of General Psychiatry, 57(4), 375–380.

Lakey, B., & Orehek, E. (2011). Relational regulation theory: A new approach to explain the link between perceived social support and mental health. Psychological Review, 118(3), 482–495.

Lovibond, S. H., & Lovibond, P. F. (1995). Manual for the Depression Anxiety Stress Scales (DASS). Psychology Foundation of Australia.

Monroe, S. M., & Harkness, K. L. (2011). Recurrence in major depression: A conceptual analysis. Psychological Review, 118(4), 655–674.

Schuch, F. B., Vancampfort, D., Firth, J., Rosenbaum, S., Ward, P. B., Silva, E. S., & Stubbs, B. (2018). Physical activity and incident depression: A meta-analysis of prospective cohort studies. American Journal of Psychiatry, 175(7), 631–648.

Segal, Z. V., Williams, J. M. G., & Teasdale, J. D. (2010). Mindfulness-based Cognitive Therapy for Depression. Guilford Press.

Stanley, B., Brown, G. K., Brent, D. A., Wells, K., Poling, K., Curry, J., & Hughes, J. (2008). Cognitive-behavioral therapy for suicide prevention (CBT-SP): Treatment model, feasibility, and acceptability. Journal of the American Academy of Child & Adolescent Psychiatry, 48(10), 1005–1013.

Wichers, M., Barge-Schaapveld, D., Nicolson, N. A., Peeters, F., de Vries, M., & van Os, J. (2011). Reduced complexity in daily life moment-to-moment variability in major depressive disorder. Behavior Research and Therapy, 49(9), 605–615.

CHAPTER 25

Spirituality and Connection

Introduction: Finding Meaning and Belonging in Recovery

For many, spirituality provides a sense of meaning, purpose, and connection that goes beyond the self, often offering unique comfort and resilience in challenging times. In the context of mental health recovery, spirituality can serve as an anchor, offering stability, inner peace, and a sense of belonging. Spirituality here is not limited to religious beliefs; it can include a broader understanding of connection to nature, personal values, or practices that build inner peace.

Depression and anxiety can create a feeling of disconnection – both from oneself and from the world. A spiritual connection, however, can bridge this gap, supporting you in finding renewed purpose, solace, and clarity. Research indicates that engaging in spiritual practices can have significant positive effects on mental health, such as reducing stress and enhancing emotional resilience (Koenig, 2012). What follows is a look at how spirituality – through practices like nature immersion, mindfulness, gratitude, and community-building – can become a sustaining resource for healing.

The Role of Spirituality in Mental Health Resilience

Spirituality can be a helpful part of a combined healing approach, helping to build acceptance, gratitude, and perspective. Here's how spirituality supports mental health resilience:

- Stress reduction: Practices like mindfulness meditation and nature immersion help ground us in the present moment, promoting relaxation and reducing cortisol levels associated with stress.

- Emotional stability: Engaging in spiritual practices often encourages reflection, self-compassion, and acceptance, which can contribute to emotional balance.

- Sense of belonging and purpose: Spirituality builds a sense of connection – whether to a community, a personal mission, or the natural world. This connection reduces feelings of loneliness and isolation, offering comfort and stability in the recovery process.

Practices for Cultivating Spirituality

- Nature immersion:
- Purpose: Nature immersion reconnects us with the world outside of ourselves, building feelings of peace, awe, and grounding. Natural settings offer a unique opportunity to fully engage our senses, creating space for mindfulness and presence.

- Instructions: Choose a natural setting that resonates with you – a park, forest, beach, or garden. As you walk or sit quietly, notice the details around you: colours, shapes, sounds, and textures. Observe without judgement, allowing each sensation to anchor you in the present.

- Mental health benefits: Immersion in nature can reduce cortisol levels, improve mood, and help alleviate symptoms of anxiety and depression. Research shows that spending even 20 minutes in nature can significantly lower stress (Bratman et al., 2019).
- Mindfulness meditation:
- Purpose: Mindfulness meditation brings our attention to the present, building awareness and acceptance of thoughts and emotions without judgement.
- Instructions: Begin by sitting in a quiet, comfortable space. Close your eyes and take deep breaths, focusing on each inhale and exhale. When your mind wanders, gently bring it back to your breath. Start with a few minutes each day, gradually increasing the time as you feel comfortable.
- Mental health benefits: Mindfulness meditation has been shown to improve emotional regulation, reduce symptoms of depression, and build resilience by helping individuals respond to stress calmly and thoughtfully (Goyal et al., 2014).
- Gratitude rituals:
- Purpose: Regular gratitude practice can shift one's focus toward the positive aspects of life, counteract negative thoughts, and promote a balanced perspective.
- Instructions: Each day, write down three things you're grateful for. These can be simple pleasures, meaningful interactions, or moments of personal insight. Reflect on each item's significance. If journaling isn't your preference, consider expressing gratitude verbally to yourself or sharing it with others.
- Mental health benefits: Regular gratitude practices are associated with improved mood, greater empathy, and reduced stress, building a strong mindset (Emmons &

Mishra, 2011).

- Finding meaning through purpose-driven activities:

- Purpose: Connecting with purpose through activities that align with your values improves fulfilment, motivation, and belonging.

- Instructions: Reflect on causes, activities, or values that hold personal meaning. Engage with these through small, intentional actions, such as volunteering, creative expression, or quality time with loved ones. Purpose-driven activities don't need to be grand; even simple actions that align with your values can bring fulfilment.

- Mental health benefits: Studies show that purpose-driven activities lead to higher life satisfaction, increased strength, and improved mental health. Engaging in meaningful activities can help build self-worth and counter feelings of isolation (Ryff & Singer, 2008).

- Expanding perspectives: exploring new faiths and building community connections:

- Purpose: Exploring new faiths and philosophies offers fresh insights into spirituality while opening doors to new communities. Meeting people with shared interests in growth can create a supportive social circle, offering a sense of belonging and camaraderie.

- Instructions: Begin with a philosophy, faith, or spiritual community that interests you, such as Buddhism, Stoicism, Indigenous spirituality, or mindfulness. Attend an open class, gathering, or group discussion, and engage with others in meaningful conversations. Reflect on your experiences and stay connected with people who resonate with you, gradually building a supportive network.

- Mental health benefits: Building a community around shared spiritual interests reduces loneliness and isolation, both everyday experiences in mental health recovery. Studies show that having a supportive social network is key to maintaining mental health and resilience (Koenig, 2012).
- Creating a personal spiritual ritual:
- Purpose: A personal ritual serves as a dedicated time each day to connect with spirituality, fostering calm reflection and emotional grounding.
- Instructions: Choose a short, meaningful activity, such as lighting a candle, reading an inspiring passage, or meditating. Set aside a few minutes each day for this ritual, using it to remind yourself of your journey and connection to something greater. Adjust your ritual as needed to reflect your evolving spiritual needs.
- Mental health benefits: Regular spiritual rituals provide a grounding anchor, reducing anxiety and promoting a sense of peace, stability, and belonging (Koenig, 2012).

The Impact of Spiritual Practices on Mental Health

Integrating spiritual practices into daily life can contribute significantly to mental health recovery by fostering inner peace, strength, and emotional stability. Spirituality can reduce stress, increase life satisfaction, and improve coping abilities for those managing depression or anxiety (Koenig, 2012). It offers perspective and helps individuals reinterpret challenges as opportunities for growth, supporting a mindset of healing and transformation in recovery.

In addition to fostering a sense of connection, spirituality provides perspective, helping individuals reframe difficult experiences. This outlook supports the goals of combined healing, building a foundation for sustained mental health.

Practical Steps to Start Your Spiritual Journey

- Experiment with different practices: Spirituality is personal; try various activities, from meditation to community involvement, and observe what resonates with you.
- Start small and consistent: Begin with a few minutes each day. Consistency is more important than duration, as even brief practices can make a meaningful difference over time.
- Reflect and adjust: Notice how different practices affect your mental state and adjust based on what brings the most peace and fulfilment.
- Seek community or guidance: Consider joining groups, taking classes, or finding a spiritual mentor. Community can provide support and deepen your sense of connection, improving the experience of spirituality.

Conclusion: Embracing Spirituality as a Source of Strength

Spirituality can be a profound source of strength, comfort, and belonging on the road to mental health recovery. By exploring diverse spiritual practices, connecting with like-minded communities, and embracing new perspectives, you create a wellspring of meaning and peace. Spiritual practices like nature immersion, gratitude, and personal rituals build inner stability and calm, while social connections through shared spiritual interests provide companionship and support.

Embrace spirituality as a personal process – one that can adapt to your needs, grow with you, and remain a source of comfort and connection. By building both inner and outer connections, spirituality supports a balanced, fulfilling recovery that extends beyond the self.

References

Bratman, G. N., Hamilton, J. P., Hahn, K. S., Daily, G. C., & Gross, J. J. (2019). Nature experience reduces rumination and subgenual prefrontal cortex activation. Proceedings of the National Academy of Sciences, 112(28), 8567–8572.

Emmons, R. A., & Mishra, A. (2011). Why gratitude improves well-being: What we know, what we need to know. In Sheldon, K. M., Kashdan, T. B., & Steger, M. F. (Eds.), Designing Positive Psychology: Taking stock and moving forward (pp. 248–262). Oxford University Press.

Goyal, M., Singh, S., Sibinga, E. M. S., Gould, N. F., Rowland-Seymour, A., Sharma, R., Berger, Z., Sleicher, D., Maron, D. D., Shihab, H. M., & Ranasinghe, P. D. (2014). Meditation programs for psychological stress and health: A systematic review and meta-analysis. JAMA Internal Medicine, 174(3), 357–368.

Koenig, H. G. (2012). Religion, Spirituality, and Health: The research and clinical implications. ISRN Psychiatry.

Ryff, C. D., & Singer, B. (2008). Know thyself and become what you are: A eudaimonic approach to psychological well-being. Journal of Happiness Studies, 9(1), 13–39.

CHAPTER 26

Forgiveness and Letting Go

Introduction: The Power of Forgiveness in Healing

Unresolved anger, bitterness, or resentment can weigh heavily on mental health, creating barriers to healing. For many, the idea of forgiveness can feel daunting or even counterproductive, especially if it seems to imply condoning hurtful actions. In this chapter, we'll redefine forgiveness as a personal, helpful choice to release emotional burdens – not to excuse or justify past wrongs. By letting go of lingering resentment and focusing on internal peace, you allow space for healing and emotional clarity. This process can be a decisive step toward mental freedom and inner balance, vital components of your combined healing process.

Exercise 1: Forgiveness Meditation

Purpose: This guided meditation helps you release resentment or anger mentally and emotionally, building compassion for yourself and others.

Instructions:

- Find a quiet space: Sit comfortably in a place where you won't be interrupted. Close your eyes and take a few deep breaths, allowing your body to relax.

- Focus on the person or situation: Gently recall the person or situation that has caused you pain. Notice any emotions that arise, acknowledging them without judgement.

- Repeat forgiveness phrases: Silently repeat phrases that resonate, such as:

- "I release the hold this pain has over me."

- "I choose peace over resentment."

- "I forgive you for my peace."

These phrases aren't about excusing what happened; instead, they are affirmations of your intention to let go of the emotional weight you carry.

- End with self-compassion: After several minutes, shift your focus back to yourself. Offer compassion and kindness for the courage it takes to forgive. Remind yourself that forgiveness is a journey and that your well-being is worth the effort.

This meditation can be revisited whenever unresolved feelings surface, allowing you to continue releasing negative emotions over time.

Exercise 2: Letter Writing (Without Sending)

Purpose: Writing an unsent letter allows you to express and release emotions safely, offering closure without needing external validation or response.

Instructions:

- Set up for honesty: Choose a time and place where you feel calm and open. Begin the letter as if you were speaking directly to the person who caused you pain.

- Express your feelings fully: write about what happened, how it affected you, and the emotions you still carry. Don't hold back – allow yourself to feel and articulate all aspects of your experience.

- Acknowledge what you're letting go: Toward the end of the letter, shift your focus to what you are ready to release. Use statements like:

- "I am letting go of this pain to free myself."

- "I choose to move forward without the weight of this resentment."

- Conclude with self-compassion: End the letter with a few words of kindness toward yourself, acknowledging the effort and strength required to forgive.

- Release the letter: You may choose to keep the letter, shred it, or burn it as a symbolic release. The act of writing and then physically releasing it can help reinforce your decision to move forward.

Exercise 3: Reframing Past Experiences

Purpose: This cognitive exercise helps you view difficult experiences from new perspectives, reducing the emotional charge they carry and building peace.

Instructions:

- Identify the situation: Choose a specific situation or experience that you struggle to forgive. Reflect on the details without judgement.

- Examine your narrative: Consider the story you tell yourself about the event. What words or phrases do you use to describe it? How does this perspective affect your emotions?

- Challenge and reframe: Gently challenge the narrative by asking questions like:

- "Is there another way to view what happened?"

- "Could I interpret this event in a way that helps me?"

- "What have I learned or gained from this experience?"

- Create a new narrative: Reframe the story to one that acknowledges the growth, resilience, or strength you've gained. For example, if you've experienced betrayal, the new narrative could emphasise how the experience taught you to set healthy boundaries and value your well-being.

This exercise may take time and repeated reflection, but each reframe gradually shifts the emotional impact of past experiences, allowing space for peace and acceptance.

The Benefits of Forgiveness in Mental Health Recovery

Forgiveness isn't just an act of kindness toward others; it is a gift to yourself. Research shows that forgiveness reduces stress levels, lowers blood pressure, and improves emotional strength (Worthington & Scherer, 2004). The process of letting go builds a state of emotional balance that supports overall mental health, aligning well with the combined healing approach. By forgiving, you free up mental and emotional energy that can be redirected toward growth, relationships, and inner peace.

Conclusion: Forgiveness as a Personal Journey

Forgiveness is not a single act but a journey of self-liberation. Each step in releasing anger, resentment, or bitterness opens space for new, positive emotions to flourish. With each practice – whether meditation, letter writing, or cognitive reframing – you move closer to a state of internal peace that supports strength, health, and self-compassion. This process of forgiveness is a profound gift to your mental health, allowing you to carry forward the wisdom and strength that emerge from letting go.

References

Enright, R. D., & Fitzgibbons, R. P. (2015). Forgiveness Therapy: An empirical guide for resolving anger and restoring hope. American Psychological Association.

Neff, K. D. (2011). Self-compassion: The proven power of being kind to yourself. William Morrow.

Seligman, M. E. P. (2011). Flourish: A visionary new understanding of happiness and well-being. Free Press.

Snyder, C. R., & Lopez, S. J. (2007). Positive Psychology: The scientific and practical explorations of human strengths (2nd ed.). Sage Publications.

Worthington, E. L., & Scherer, M. (2004). Forgiveness is an emotion-focused coping strategy that can reduce health risks and promote health resilience: Theory, review, and hypotheses. Psychology & Health, 19(3), 385–405.

CHAPTER 27

The Role of Gratitude and Positive Psychology in Recovery

Introduction: Embracing Positivity in the Recovery Journey

Positive psychology, the study of human strengths, virtues, and positive emotions, offers practical tools for improving strength and supporting mental health recovery. Traditional mental health approaches focus primarily on alleviating symptoms, but positive psychology encourages the cultivation of strengths like gratitude, optimism, kindness, and meaning. Shifting focus from what's difficult to what's thriving can strengthen stability and bring balance to your healing journey. In this chapter, we'll explore the role of gratitude, optimism, and other positive psychology practices, providing practical ways to build well-being and support long-term recovery.

Understanding Positive Psychology in Depression Recovery

Positive psychology's emphasis on positive emotions and personal strengths has shown significant benefits for mental health recovery. Research suggests that intentionally cultivating positive experiences and mindsets can help improve mood, motivation, and strength:

- The science of positive emotions: Positive emotions like gratitude, joy, and hope support neuroplasticity – the brain's ability to create new neural pathways (Fredrickson, 2001). This adaptability helps interrupt cycles of negative thinking and supports cognitive flexibility.

- Improved health and motivation: Positive practices such as gratitude journaling or acts of kindness have been shown to increase life satisfaction and decrease symptoms of depression (Emmons & McCullough, 2003). These practices can help shift focus from challenges to achievements, sustaining motivation in recovery.

- Building strength: Positive psychology fosters strength by reinforcing self-worth and building coping skills. Developing strengths and focusing on positive experiences can build a solid emotional foundation, helping individuals better handle setbacks and challenges.

The Benefits of Practicing Gratitude

Gratitude is a core component of positive psychology, and it provides a wealth of mental health benefits. Regularly practising gratitude helps shift attention toward the positives, buffers against negative thoughts, and reduces stress.

- Enhanced happiness and life satisfaction: Research shows that gratitude can increase happiness and life satisfaction by up to 25% (Seligman et al., 2005). This practice helps reinforce positive experiences, creating a more balanced perspective.

- Reduced stress and improved emotional regulation: Expressing gratitude can lower cortisol levels and promote relaxation, helping to manage stress (Sansone & Sansone, 2010). Practising gratitude helps regulate emotions, reducing the intensity of anxiety or depressive symptoms.
- Strengthened social bonds: Expressing gratitude strengthens relationships by increasing trust and appreciation. Strong relationships play an essential role in recovery, reducing feelings of isolation and providing support (Algoe et al., 2010).

Integrating Positive Psychology Practices into Daily Life

Positive psychology offers many practical tools that you can incorporate into daily routines to enhance health. These practices help establish a routine of positivity that supports both immediate mood improvements and long-term strength.

1. Gratitude journaling

Each day, write down three things you're grateful for, no matter how small. Studies show that this practice can increase life satisfaction, improve mood, and reduce depressive symptoms (Emmons & McCullough, 2003).
Example: "I'm grateful for the walk I took in the park, the kindness of a friend, and the delicious meal I had for dinner."

2. Acts of kindness

Performing acts of kindness – helping a friend, volunteering, or offering a compliment – builds connection and provides a sense of purpose. Acts of kindness can increase happiness and health, and they counter feelings of isolation (Curry et al., 2018).

Example: Aim to do one act of kindness each day, whether it's holding the door open for someone or sending a thoughtful text to a loved one.

3. Savouring Positive Experiences

Savouring is the practice of fully immersing yourself in positive moments, amplifying their impact on mood and memory. Studies show that savouring can improve mood, reduce stress, and create lasting positive memories (Bryant & Veroff, 2007).

Example: When drinking your morning coffee, take time to focus on its warmth, aroma, and taste. Be present in the moment and appreciate it fully.

4. Self-Compassion and Positive Affirmations

Practising self-compassion involves treating yourself with kindness and understanding, especially when facing challenges. Positive affirmations help reinforce self-worth and improve resilience (Critcher & Dunning, 2015).

Example: When you catch yourself thinking critically, counter it with a compassionate statement, such as, "I'm doing my best, and that's enough."

5. Expressing Gratitude to Others

Expressing gratitude to others can boost feelings of connection and increase positive emotions. Taking time to thank others reinforces social bonds, which are critical for recovery.

Example: Write a note of thanks to someone who has had a positive impact on your life. Even if you don't send it, this practice can strengthen your focus on meaningful relationships.

The Power of Optimism in Recovery

Optimism – expecting positive outcomes – can improve strength and help individuals approach life's challenges with a growth mindset. Optimism doesn't ignore difficulties but instead views them as surmountable, building an attitude of hopefulness that supports recovery.

Optimistic individuals experience better physical health, higher life satisfaction, and stronger resilience (Carver et al., 2010). Optimism in recovery supports adaptability and helps counter negative self-talk.

To build optimism, reframe negative thoughts, visualise positive outcomes, and set realistic, hopeful goals. These strategies reinforce an expectation of success, which strengthens motivation and confidence.

Flow and Engagement in Meaningful Activities

Flow is a state of complete engagement in an activity. When in this state, you feel focused and absorbed, losing track of time. Flow experiences boost mood, support a sense of purpose, and build health.

Engaging in flow activities can improve mood, reduce symptoms of depression, and increase motivation (Csikszentmihalyi, 1990). In recovery, flow can serve as a reminder of your capacity for joy and engagement.

Identify activities that make you lose track of time, such as playing music, painting, or gardening. Incorporating flow experiences into your weekly routine adds balance and satisfaction.

Meaning and Purpose in Recovery

Finding meaning and purpose contributes significantly to mental health, giving life a sense of direction and connection. People with a strong sense of purpose often report lower stress levels and greater life satisfaction, making purpose-driven activities valuable in recovery (Ryff, 1989).

Identify causes, hobbies, or activities that feel meaningful. This could be volunteering, creating art, or pursuing a spiritual practice – anything that aligns with your values and interests.

Building Emotional Intelligence

Emotional Intelligence (EI) includes skills like self-awareness, self-regulation, and empathy. Developing EI strengthens emotional strength and promotes healthier social interactions. Higher EI is associated with better stress management, lower rates of depression, and improved relationships (Goleman, 1995).

Reflect on your emotional responses, practice empathy, and regulate reactions to stressful situations. Mindfulness and journaling can also improve emotional intelligence over time.

Positive Relationships as a Foundation for Recovery

Positive relationships provide emotional support and social connection, which are essential for mental health. Investing in supportive relationships builds a stable foundation for long-term recovery.

Make time for uplifting and supportive relationships. Communicate appreciation and practice active listening to deepen connections. When someone shares good news, respond with interest and enthusiasm. This practice, known as active constructive responding, fosters closer relationships and increases happiness (Gable et al., 2004).

Key Takeaways

- Gratitude and optimism improve strength: Regularly practising gratitude and optimism strengthens your ability to handle challenges.

- Flow activities bring purpose: Activities that engage you fully build focus, enjoyment, and satisfaction.

- Emotional intelligence improves coping skills: Practicing EI supports emotional regulation and strengthens social connections.

- Positive relationships build stability: Investing in strong, supportive relationships reinforces resilience and reduces isolation.

Conclusion: Building Positivity into Daily Life

Positive psychology practices don't replace the hard work of recovery; they improve it, providing tools to support strength and well-being. By incorporating gratitude, optimism, purpose, and positive social connections into daily life, you build a solid foundation for mental health. These practices build self-compassion, stability, and motivation, helping you move forward with confidence and optimism.

References

Algoe, S. B., Haidt, J., & Gable, S. L. (2010). Beyond reciprocity: Gratitude and relationships in everyday life. Emotion, 10(1), 38–48.

Bryant, F. B., & Veroff, J. (2007). Savoring: A new model of positive experience. Psychology Press.

Carver, C. S., Scheier, M. F., & Segerstrom, S. C. (2010). Optimism. Clinical Psychology Review, 30(7), 879–889.

Critcher, C. R., & Dunning, D. (2015). Self-affirmations provide a broader perspective on self-threat. Personality and Social Psychology Bulletin, 41(1), 3–18.

Csikszentmihalyi, M. (1990). Flow: The psychology of optimal experience. Harper & Row.

Curry, O. S., Rowland, L. A., Zlotowitz, S., McAlaney, J., & Whitehouse, H. (2018). Happy to help? A systematic review and meta-analysis of the effects of performing acts of kindness on the well-being of the actor. Journal of Experimental Social Psychology, 76, 320–329.

Emmons, R. A., & McCullough, M. E. (2003). Counting blessings versus burdens: An experimental investigation of gratitude and subjective well-being in daily life. Journal of Personality and Social Psychology, 84(2), 377–389.

Fredrickson, B. L. (2001). The role of positive emotions in positive psychology: The broaden-and-build theory of positive emotions. American Psychologist, 56(3), 218–226.

Gable, S. L., Reis, H. T., Impett, E. A., & Asher, E. R. (2004). What do you do when things go right? The intrapersonal and interpersonal benefits of sharing positive events. Journal of Personality and Social Psychology, 87(2), 228–245.

Goleman, D. (1995). Emotional Intelligence. Bantam Books.

McCraty, R., & Childre, D. (2004). The grateful heart: The psychophysiology of appreciation. The Humanistic Psychologist, 32(3), 26–45.

Ryff, C. D. (1989). Happiness is everything, or is it? Explorations on the meaning of psychological well-being. Journal of Personality and Social Psychology, 57(6), 1069–1081.

Sansone, R. A., & Sansone, L. A. (2010). Gratitude and well being: The benefits of appreciation. Psychiatry, 7(11), 18–22.

Seligman, M. E. P., Steen, T. A., Park, N., & Peterson, C. (2005). Positive psychology progress: Empirical validation of interventions. American Psychologist, 60(5), 410–421.

CHAPTER 28

Exploring Identity Beyond Depression

Introduction: Rediscovering the Self Beyond Illness

Depression can cast a shadow over one's sense of self, often making it difficult to see oneself as anything other than the symptoms and limitations associated with the condition. For many, the experience of living with depression may leave their interests, hobbies, and ambitions sidelined or forgotten. This chapter is about rediscovering who you are beyond depression. Reconnecting with values, goals, and passions can be a profound motivator in recovery and a meaningful way to re-establish a fulfilling, purposeful life. You are more than your depression, and this chapter will guide you in uncovering what brings you joy, purpose, and meaning.

Exercise 1: Value-Setting and Strength Discovery

Purpose: This exercise helps you identify core values and strengths, serving as guiding lights in your journey of rediscovery and renewal.

Instructions:

- Identify core values: Review the following list of values and select the ones that resonate with you: compassion, creativity, curiosity, integrity, kindness, perseverance, relationships, security, self-expression, spirituality, wisdom. Feel free to add any values that are not listed here but hold personal significance.

- Reflect on past experiences: Write down three to five moments in your life when you felt most fulfilled, proud, or connected to your values. Reflect on questions like:

- What were you doing?

- What values were you honouring?

- How did this experience make you feel about yourself?

- Explore your strengths: Reflect on strengths you may have demonstrated during these experiences, such as courage, patience, humour, or adaptability. By identifying these values and strengths, you build a clearer understanding of the qualities that make you uniquely you, regardless of depression.

Exercise 2: Imagining a Fulfilling Future

Purpose: This exercise encourages you to visualise a future that aligns with your values and aspirations, helping you define meaningful goals.

Instructions:

- Reflect on your ideal day: Take a few moments to write down what an ideal day would look like if you felt fully connected to your values and goals. Consider:

- How would you start your day?

- What activities would you prioritise?

- Who would you spend time with, and how would these relationships support your health?
- Identify key aspects of fulfilment: From your description of an ideal day, highlight specific activities or qualities that feel most fulfilling to you. These might include creativity, connection, physical well-being, or quiet reflection.
- Set a few meaningful goals: Based on these reflections, create a list of three to five small goals or actions that bring you closer to this vision. For example:
- If the connection feels essential, you might aim to schedule regular time with friends.
- If you value personal growth, set aside a few hours each week to learn a new skill.
- Revisit your ideal day: Over time, revisit and adjust this vision as your understanding of fulfilment grows. This will help you stay aligned with what genuinely matters to you.

Exercise 3: Life Purpose Mapping

Purpose: Life purpose mapping helps to explore the "why" behind your goals, adding a sense of purpose and fulfilment to your journey.

Instructions:

- Reflect on impact and fulfilment: Consider these prompts and jot down your thoughts:
- If I could make a difference in one area of life, what would it be?
- What brings me a deep sense of fulfilment, regardless of how big or small?
- Define purpose in daily actions: Based on these reflections, think about daily or weekly actions that align with this

purpose. For example:

- If connection brings fulfilment, consider setting a goal to call or meet a friend each week.
- If creativity is meaningful, schedule regular time to write, draw, or engage in another creative pursuit.
- Revisit periodically: Life purpose mapping is a dynamic process. As your goals and interests evolve, revisit and revise this map periodically.

Reflective Exercise: The Future Self-Letter

Purpose: Writing a letter from your future self serves as a source of motivation and hope, helping you to imagine a life enriched by self-fulfilment.

Instructions:

- Imagine your future self: Picture yourself a few years from now, having made progress toward your goals and strengthened your sense of identity.
- Write a letter: From this perspective, write a letter to your current self, reflecting on:
- How you overcame setbacks.
- What you are grateful for in your journey.
- Words of encouragement and advice that would have helped you along the way.
- Keep and reflect: Keep this letter and read it whenever you need a reminder of the potential for a future that includes growth, fulfilment, and stability beyond depression.

Conclusion: The Ongoing Journey of Self-Discovery

Reclaiming your identity and building a life of purpose is an ongoing process. Just as you are more than your depression, your identity will continue to grow and evolve. This chapter's exercises – value-setting, imagining a fulfilling future, life purpose mapping, and the future self-letter – can serve as tools to explore your identity over time. By reconnecting with your values and passions, you can envision and work toward a life that feels authentic, fulfilling, and truly yours.

References

Neff, K. D. (2011). Self-compassion: The proven power of being kind to yourself. William Morrow.

Rubin, G. (2015). Better Than Before: Mastering the habits of our everyday lives. Crown Publishing Group.

Seligman, M. E. P. (2011). Flourish: A visionary new understanding of happiness and well-being. Free Press.

Snyder, C. R., & Lopez, S. J. (2007). Positive Psychology: The scientific and practical explorations of human strengths (2nd ed.). Sage Publications.

Van der Kolk, B. (2014). The Body Keeps the Score: Brain, mind, and body in the healing of trauma. Viking.

CHAPTER 29

Building Emotional Intelligence for Mental Resilience

Introduction: The Role of Emotions in Mental Health and Resilience

Emotions are integral to the human experience, acting as an internal guidance system to help us respond to our environment, connect with others, and make decisions. Emotional Intelligence (EI) involves recognising, understanding, and managing these emotions effectively. By developing EI, we gain the tools to navigate life's challenges, deepen relationships, and build strength. In mental health recovery, EI becomes essential for building self-awareness, emotional stability, and personal growth within a combined healing approach.

Why Do We Have Emotions?

From an evolutionary standpoint, emotions evolved to guide us in surviving and thriving in a complex world. Emotions such as fear, joy, anger, and sadness serve essential functions:

- Survival and safety: Emotions like fear alert us to danger, preparing the body for fight-or-flight. Anger, when appropriate, motivates us to defend our boundaries. These emotions kept our ancestors alert to potential threats.

- Connection and social bonds: Emotions such as love, empathy, and gratitude foster cooperation and trust, strengthening social bonds. Positive emotions encourage relationships and mutual support, which is important in societies where interdependence is a core survival strategy.

- Decision-making and learning: Emotions guide our decisions by indicating what aligns or conflicts with our values, goals, or needs. For example, feelings of discomfort might prompt us to reassess a situation, while joy and satisfaction signal alignment with our goals.

- Personal growth and adaptation: Emotions also drive learning and adaptation. After setbacks, emotions like disappointment or sadness lead to self-reflection, prompting changes that build personal growth.

Understanding the purpose of emotions helps us view them as signals rather than obstacles. Emotions, when acknowledged and managed effectively, can be powerful allies in navigating life's complexities.

The Value of Emotional Intelligence

Emotional Intelligence (EI) builds on our natural emotional responses, enabling us to understand, process, and use them constructively. Rather than being controlled by emotions, EI helps us to respond with clarity and resilience. In a combined healing approach, EI improves each layer by:

- Managing stress and responding flexibly: EI builds self-regulation, helping us manage challenging emotions constructively. This is critical for handling stress, particularly when adjusting to new lifestyle layers like nutrition, sleep, or exercise.

- Building strength: Recognising that emotions are temporary and often tied to immediate factors strengthens resilience. EI enables us to acknowledge emotions, respond constructively, and adapt, even in difficult moments.

- Enhancing social connections and support systems: EI improves empathy and social awareness, allowing us to express our emotions accurately to others. When we communicate emotions clearly – like saying, "I feel anxious and could use some reassurance" – it invites understanding and compassion from friends, family, or caregivers. This open communication strengthens support networks, which are important in combined healing.

- Promoting self-awareness and personal growth: EI deepens self-awareness, encouraging us to observe our emotional responses and understand their roots. This leads to a more authentic, adaptable way of engaging with life, improving growth and healing.

The pages ahead cover the four components of EI – self-awareness, self-regulation, social awareness, and relationship management – along with practical exercises. Understanding and building EI helps us to interpret and communicate our emotions effectively, creating a solid foundation for strength in combined healing.

The Components of Emotional Intelligence

Self-Awareness: The Foundation of Emotional Intelligence

Self-awareness is the foundation of EI. It allows us to recognise and understand our emotions and how they shape our thoughts and behaviours. It also includes recognising how physical states, such as blood sugar levels, sleep quality, and stress hormones, impact emotions. Realising that emotions are often temporary responses to specific factors can help us approach them with flexibility, self-compassion, and mindfulness.

Steps to cultivate self-awareness include:

• Mindful journaling: Reflect on your emotions daily, noting the events, interactions, and physical factors that triggered them. This practice reveals patterns, showing that emotions often arise from specific triggers and reinforcing the idea that they are temporary.

• Daily emotional check-ins: Ask yourself regularly, "What am I feeling right now?" and "What might be causing these feelings?" Observing emotions as they fluctuate day to day reinforces that emotions are often responses to immediate circumstances.

• Identifying core beliefs and temporary triggers: Recognising which beliefs or physical factors affect emotions helps differentiate deeper emotional triggers from fleeting reactions, building a balanced view of emotional states.

Self-Awareness Exercise: Emotion Labelling

When experiencing a strong emotion, label it specifically. Instead of "I'm upset", try "I feel disappointed" or "I'm frustrated". Studies show that labelling emotions reduces their intensity by up to 30% and reinforces that emotions are manageable responses to specific situations (Lieberman et al., 2007).

Self-Regulation: Managing Emotions Constructively

Self-regulation is the ability to manage emotions constructively, even when physical or environmental factors heighten them. This skill allows us to pause, reflect, and respond thoughtfully, helping to prevent impulsive reactions. Recognising that emotions can shift over time supports the practice of responding calmly, knowing that strong feelings often change. Self-regulation can reduce symptoms of anxiety and depression, contributing to mental strength by 15-20% (Gross, 2002).

Steps to practice self-regulation include:

- Breathing techniques: Techniques like the "4-7-8" breath activate the body's relaxation response, helping calm both mind and body. Knowing that intentional breathing can shift emotional states makes it an invaluable self-regulation tool.

- Pause and reflect: When a strong emotion arises, pause before reacting. This brief break allows you to observe and understand the emotion, acknowledging that its intensity may decrease with time.

- Self-soothing techniques: Develop a toolkit of self-soothing methods, such as music, grounding exercises, or visualisation, to manage emotions. Self-soothing not only calms the body but reinforces the knowledge that emotions can change with intentional practices.

Self-Regulation Exercise: The Five-Second Rule

When faced with an emotionally charged situation, count down from five before reacting. This activates decision-making centres in the brain, helping you respond with intention (Robbins, 2017).

Social Awareness: Building Empathy and Understanding

Social awareness involves empathising with others and understanding that their emotions are also influenced by various factors. Recognising the dynamic nature of emotions builds empathy and builds stronger connections. This understanding enables us to communicate our own emotions clearly and invite understanding from others, which is particularly valuable in creating a supportive network. High social awareness can increase relationship satisfaction by up to 30% (Davis, 1983).

Steps to improve social awareness include:

- Active listening: Practise active listening by fully focusing on the speaker and avoiding interruptions. This approach helps you understand others' emotions more clearly and invites similar understanding from them.

- Reading nonverbal cues: Observing body language, facial expressions, and tone helps you understand others' emotions and provides insight into how best to respond with empathy.

- Empathy exercises: Practice perspective-taking by imagining yourself in someone else's situation. This builds empathy and builds supportive connections by acknowledging that others' feelings, too, are subject to change.

Social Awareness Exercise: Empathy Mapping

During interactions, consider what the other person might be thinking, feeling, saying, and doing. This exercise builds a fuller understanding of others' emotions and reminds you that feelings are often responses to particular situations.

Relationship Management: Strengthening Connections

Relationship management helps you build and sustain a network of supportive relationships that build resilience.

Understanding that emotions are dynamic can help us approach relationships with flexibility, patience, and empathy. Additionally, being able to communicate our own emotions clearly encourages those around us to understand and support us. In mental health recovery, relationship management provides stability, reducing isolation and reinforcing strength.

Steps to develop relationship management skills include:

- Effective communication: Use "I" statements to express feelings respectfully and clearly. Open communication helps build trust and understanding, especially when acknowledging that emotions often change.

- Conflict resolution: Approach conflicts constructively, knowing that emotions experienced during conflict are often temporary. Constructive conflict resolution strengthens relationships and creates long-lasting bonds.

- Showing appreciation: Express gratitude to those around you. Recognising others' support and contributions builds solid relationships and a stable support system.

Relationship Management Exercise: Weekly Appreciation Check-In

Express appreciation to someone in your life each week. This simple act strengthens connections, reinforces your support network, and builds emotional resilience.

Practical Routine for Building Emotional Intelligence

Integrate these EI practices into daily life, reinforcing that emotions are temporary and valuable responses to various influences:

- Morning: Start with a few minutes of mindfulness to cultivate self-awareness, observing any initial emotional states.

- During the day: Practise active listening, empathy mapping, and emotion labelling. Notice how emotions change in response to different situations.

- Evening: Reflect on any intense emotions from the day, label them, and journal about how they evolved or subsided. Recognising these patterns reinforces the understanding that emotions shift.

This routine supports self-awareness, self-regulation, social awareness, and relationship management, building a balanced, strong foundation for mental health recovery.

How Emotional Intelligence Supports a Layered Healing Approach

In a combined healing approach, EI enhances each component of recovery:

- Self-awareness as a foundation for all layers: Self-awareness helps individuals connect physical health (sleep, nutrition, exercise) with emotional states, reinforcing the effects of each base layer in recovery.

- Self-regulation to improve coping mechanisms: Self-regulation supports stress management techniques across layers, ensuring consistent progress without emotional setbacks.

- Social awareness to strengthen support systems: Social awareness and empathy build supportive, understanding relationships that strengthen each healing layer, particularly by improving communication with friends, family, and caregivers.

- Relationship management as a layer for sustained progress: Healthy relationships reduce isolation and create an additional support layer, reinforcing progress in recovery.

- Adapting to changes in each layer: Recognising emotions as fluid responses to change helps individuals stay flexible and committed to recovery.

By layering EI with foundational practices, individuals create a balanced, strong approach to recovery that supports mental wellness and builds long-term stability.

CHAPTER 30

Advanced Integrative Techniques for Mental Health

Introduction: Integrating Body and Mind for Holistic Healing

Advanced integrative techniques extend beyond conventional approaches by addressing both physical and mental aspects of well-being, supporting strength, emotional stability, and self-regulation. This chapter looks at a range of powerful tools – such as nootropics, amino acids, herbs, peptides, and other techniques – that harness the body's natural processes to support brain function, mood, and stress stability. These methods complement other therapeutic approaches, creating a thorough, adaptive healing framework.

The Science of Advanced Integrative Techniques

1. Nootropics

Nootropics are compounds that improve cognitive function, improve memory, and support mental clarity. They can be natural or synthetic compounds that benefit brain health. Nootropics are often referred to as "smart drugs".

- Science and research: Certain nootropics, such as lion's mane, bacopa monnieri, and ginkgo biloba, are linked to improved cognitive performance and reduced symptoms of anxiety or depression (McGreevy et al., 2016).
- Practical application: For brain support, start with natural nootropics like lion's mane mushroom or bacopa. Incorporate them daily in capsule or tea form for enhanced focus and mental clarity.

2. Amino Acids and Peptides

Amino acids are essential for neurotransmitter production and overall brain function. Peptides, which are short chains of amino acids, can support mood, energy, and recovery. Specific peptides specifically aid brain health.

- Science and research: Amino acids like L-tyrosine support dopamine production, helping with focus and energy, while L-theanine supports calmness. Peptides like BPC-157 have shown anti-inflammatory properties in animal studies (Smith et al., 2020). However, it is important to note that there are currently zero published human clinical trials examining BPC-157 for psychiatric conditions. Additionally, because BPC-157 promotes angiogenesis (new blood vessel formation), there are theoretical safety concerns regarding the potential acceleration of undiagnosed tumour growth. In early 2026, U.S. regulatory discussions proposed moving BPC-157 from the FDA's restricted Category 2 list back to Category 1, restoring legal access through prescription compounding — but this does not constitute FDA or TGA approval. BPC-157 should be treated as highly experimental.
- Practical application: Amino acids can be taken as supplements to support specific neurotransmitters. For peptides such as BPC-157 or Semax, consult a healthcare provider before considering any peptide therapy. Given the

lack of human clinical trial data for psychiatric use and the theoretical safety concerns around angiogenesis, peptide therapies should only be explored under close medical supervision.

3. Herbs for Cognitive and Emotional Support

For centuries, herbs have been used to support mood, energy, and mental clarity. Adaptogens, in particular, are herbs that help the body adapt to stress.

- Science and research: Herbs like ashwagandha, rhodiola, and holy basil reduce cortisol levels and support emotional strength by modulating the stress response (Panossian et al., 2017).
- Practical application: Adaptogenic herbs can be taken as teas, tinctures, or capsules. Start with ashwagandha or rhodiola for stress relief and energy balance, incorporating them into your daily routine.

4. Methylation Support

Methylation is a biochemical process essential for brain health. It involves activating molecules that support neurotransmitter production, DNA repair, and detoxification. Impaired methylation is linked to mood disorders, brain fog, and fatigue.

- Science and research: Supporting methylation through B vitamins, especially B6, B12, and folate, improves neurotransmitter production and reduces homocysteine levels, which are associated with cognitive decline (Krebs et al., 2013).
- Practical application: Methylated B vitamins, such as methyl folate and methylcobalamin, can support mental clarity and

mood. Testing for methylation markers may provide insights into personalised supplementation needs.

5. Ketosis and Brain Health

Ketosis is a metabolic state where the body burns fat for fuel, producing ketones that serve as an alternative energy source for the brain. Ketogenic diets, or periods of intermittent fasting, can support cognitive clarity and mood stability.

- Science and research: Ketones are an efficient brain fuel, reducing oxidative stress and supporting mitochondrial health. Clinical trials show mixed but promising results: the 2025 KIND trial reported a 59–71% decrease in depression scores among adherent participants, while the 2026 DIME trial (JAMA Psychiatry) found initial improvements that faded by 12 weeks without intensive support. A 2026 modified Delphi consensus of international experts established the first formalised framework for using Ketogenic Metabolic Therapy (KMT) in adults with serious mood disorders, officially recognising it as a biologically plausible intervention. Long-term adherence remains the main challenge.
- Practical application: Begin with intermittent fasting or a low-carb ketogenic diet, gradually adjusting based on your energy and mental clarity. Ketone supplements are also available for a faster boost in cognitive performance.

6. Infrared Sauna Therapy

Infrared sauna therapy uses infrared light to heat the body, supporting detoxification, reducing inflammation, and enhancing relaxation. It supports the mind-body connection by alleviating physical and mental stress.

- Science and research: Regular sauna use reduces cortisol levels, increases circulation, and improves the release of endorphins, providing mood-lifting effects. Research suggests that saunas can reduce depressive symptoms and improve sleep (Laukkanen et al., 2018).
- Practical application: Start with 10–15 minutes per session, two to three times a week, gradually increasing as tolerated. Sauna therapy can improve mental clarity and relaxation, especially when paired with hydration.

Additional Integrative Techniques

Heart Rate Variability (HRV) Biofeedback

HRV biofeedback measures variations in heart rate, providing insight into autonomic nervous system function. HRV biofeedback is particularly useful for managing stress and improving strength.

- Science and research: HRV biofeedback improves emotional regulation and reduces stress by increasing parasympathetic activity. Studies show it can improve strength and reduce anxiety (Lehrer & Gevirtz, 2020).
- Practical application: Practice using HRV apps or biofeedback devices for 10–20 minutes daily, gradually increasing emotional stability and strength.

Cold Water Therapy (Cryotherapy)

Cold water therapy involves short-term cold exposure to stimulate the vagus nerve and support strength. It triggers the body's natural stress response, improving mood and emotional regulation.

- Science and research: Cold exposure triggers endorphins and reduces inflammation, positively affecting mood. Cold therapy may alleviate symptoms of depression and anxiety by improving stress strength (Shevchuk, 2008).
- Practical application: Begin with 30 seconds to 1 minute of cold water exposure, such as cold showers, and gradually increase the duration.

Acupuncture

Acupuncture balances energy by inserting thin needles into specific points on the body, which is effective for anxiety, mood regulation, and PTSD symptom relief.

- Science and research: Acupuncture modulates neurotransmitters and reduces inflammation, supporting relaxation. Studies suggest it improves mood through endorphin release and regulation of stress hormones (Wang et al., 2013).
- Practical application: Acupuncture sessions typically last 30–60 minutes, and regular sessions can help with emotional regulation and stress relief.

Biofeedback therapy

Biofeedback uses sensors to monitor physiological responses, such as muscle tension, to increase awareness and control over autonomic functions and reduce stress.

- Science and research: Biofeedback supports emotional regulation by providing physiological feedback. It has been shown to reduce anxiety and improve focus (Yu et al., 2018).
- Practical application: Home biofeedback devices or professional sessions provide training for 15–30 minutes daily, helping modulate physiological responses to stress.

Kundalini Yoga

Kundalini yoga combines breathwork, meditation, and physical movement to stimulate the nervous system, increase awareness, and balance energy and mood.

- Science and research: Kundalini yoga reduces symptoms of anxiety and depression by regulating cortisol and improving awareness. Research shows it can improve mood and reduce stress by up to 30% (Shannahoff-Khalsa, 2013).

- Practical application: Practice Kundalini yoga two to three times weekly to regulate mood and energy. Incorporate breathing exercises, postures, and meditation.

How Advanced Integrative Techniques Amplify Other Healing Layers

- Enhanced emotional and cognitive regulation: Techniques like HRV biofeedback, neuroacoustic therapy, and tDCS help stabilise emotions by inducing calm brain states and improving neuronal communication. These benefits support cognitive therapies, increasing focus and emotional engagement.

- Improved physical resilience: Techniques such as infrared sauna, ketogenic diet, and hydrogen therapy reduce oxidative stress and neuroinflammation, supporting resilience and improving engagement in daily routines and physical activity.

- Increased mindfulness and body awareness: Practices like Kundalini yoga, biofeedback, and forest bathing increase awareness of physiological rhythms, support mindfulness and prevent emotional overwhelm.

References

Krebs, M. O., Guillin, O., & Bourdel, M.-C. (2013). The importance of methylation in neuropsychiatric disorders. Current Psychiatry Reports, 15(6), Article 375. https://doi.org/10.1007/s11920-013-0375-4

Laukkanen, T., Kunutsor, S. K., Kauhanen, J., & Laukkanen, J. A. (2018). Association between sauna bathing and mental health: A cross-sectional study. Mayo Clinic Proceedings, 93(5), 634–642. https://doi.org/10.1016/j.mayocp.2018.01.034

Lehrer, P. M., & Gevirtz, R. (2020). Heart rate variability biofeedback: How and why does it work? Frontiers in Psychology, 11, Article 756. https://doi.org/10.3389/fpsyg.2020.00756

Panossian, A., & Wikman, G. (2017). Effects of adaptogens on the central nervous system and the molecular mechanisms associated with their stress-protective activity. Pharmaceuticals, 3(1), 188–224. https://doi.org/10.3390/ph30010018

CHAPTER 31

Summary of Core Healing Principles

Introduction: Embracing a Lifelong Journey of Healing

Recovery is not a fixed destination but an evolving process that calls for gentle maintenance, adaptability, and self-compassion. This chapter unites the principles from each part of the combined healing approach into a roadmap for lifelong strength, growth, and mental wellness. As you continue this journey, these core principles will serve as guides to prevent relapse, maintain mental balance, and build ongoing healing and fulfilment.

Core Principles for Lasting Mental Health

1. Laying the Foundations of Physical Well-Being

- Core chapters: Sleep (Chapter 3), Exercise and Movement (Chapter 5), Nutrition (Chapter 4), Blood Sugar Regulation (Chapter 6).
- Key elements: Prioritise restful sleep, balanced nutrition, regular movement, and stable blood sugar.
- Summary: Physical health practices create a strong base that supports all other healing layers. Regular sleep, exercise, and

balanced nutrition reduce inflammation, boost mood, and support strength. Blood sugar regulation further stabilises energy levels and helps prevent mood swings.

- Ongoing practices: Maintain a routine that respects these foundational needs – getting adequate sleep, moving daily, and eating well-balanced meals. This physical foundation provides stability that improves emotional strength and supports mental health.

2. Aligning with Natural Rhythms and Environment

- Core chapters: Sunlight, Breathwork, Circadian Rhythms, and Grounding, Environmental Detox

- Key elements: Exposure to natural light, grounding, regulated circadian rhythms, and minimising environmental toxins.

- Summary: Natural alignment with environmental cues, such as sunlight and fresh air, helps regulate mood and energy. Detoxifying your surroundings by reducing exposure to toxins and increasing access to fresh air supports mental clarity and physical well-being.

- Ongoing practices: Prioritise daily sunlight, grounding practices, and breathwork, while minimising exposure to synthetic toxins. Simple adjustments like walking outdoors, breathing deeply, and opening windows can keep you connected to nature and support a calm, centred mindset.

3. Nurturing Gut Health for Mental Balance

- Core chapter: Gut Health and Mental Wellness.

- Key elements: Balanced gut microbiome through diet, fasting, and probiotic-rich foods.

- Summary: Gut health is directly linked to mental well-being through the gut-brain axis. A balanced microbiome supports the production of neurotransmitters that regulate mood.

- Ongoing practices: Incorporate gut-friendly foods, consider fasting if it suits your body, and focus on fresh, minimally processed foods. Small, consistent efforts in gut health support both physical vitality and mental stability.

4. Finding the Right Therapeutic Approaches

- Core chapter: Discovering the Right Psychotherapy for Your Recovery.
- Key elements: Evidence-based therapies like CBT, EMDR, and somatic therapy, alongside alternatives like Gestalt, family constellations, and equine therapy.
- Summary: Therapy offers tools for processing emotions, trauma, and thoughts. The right therapeutic approach can be transformative, providing methods to navigate complex emotions and support healing.
- Ongoing practices: Choose a therapy that aligns with your needs, and stay engaged with the process. Regular check-ins with a therapist can reinforce emotional regulation skills, helping prevent relapse and building mental strength.

5. Developing Emotional Resilience and Self-Compassion

- Core chapters: Memory Integration, Beyond the Therapy Session – Living Your Psychotherapy Skills.
- Key elements: Integrating therapy skills into daily life, managing triggers, cultivating self-compassion.
- Summary: Emotional strength and self-compassion are cultivated through the skills learned in therapy, including memory processing, self-soothing, and developing healthy coping mechanisms. These tools allow you to navigate life's ups and downs with greater balance.
- Ongoing practices: Practice self-compassion and actively apply therapy skills daily. Journaling, mindfulness, and

regular self-check-ins help sustain emotional stability and prevent emotional overwhelm.

6. Practising Mindful Digital Consumption

- Core chapter: Digital Detox and Media Consumption.
- Key elements: Limiting screen time, curating positive influences, and setting boundaries with technology.
- Summary: Mindful digital habits reduce mental clutter and lower stress associated with constant online engagement. Limiting notifications and reducing screen time can improve focus, enhance mood, and support mental clarity.
- Ongoing practices: Set screen-free times, unfollow negative influences, and engage in regular digital detoxes. Creating digital boundaries builds a more present and peaceful mind, contributing to long-term mental well-being.

7. Fostering Spirituality and Connection

- Core chapter: Spirituality and Connection.
- Key elements: Personal spiritual practices, gratitude, nature immersion, and building a spiritual community.
- Summary: Spiritual practices offer comfort, purpose, and a sense of connection. Whether through mindfulness, nature, or meaningful community involvement, spirituality provides inner peace and a sense of belonging.
- Ongoing practices: Integrate mindfulness, gratitude rituals, and spiritual reflection into your daily routine. Engaging with like-minded communities can reinforce a sense of purpose and foster strength in challenging times.

8. Building Emotional Intelligence and Connection

- Core chapter: Building Emotional Intelligence for Mental Resilience.

- Key elements: Awareness of emotions, empathy, self-regulation, and social support.
- Summary: Emotional intelligence improves your capacity to understand, express, and manage emotions. Recognising and addressing emotions as they arise strengthens relationships and improves coping skills.
- Ongoing practices: Develop emotional awareness through regular self-reflection and mindfulness. Embrace social support and practice empathy in interactions, reinforcing both personal and relational strength.

9. Exploring Identity Beyond Depression

- Core chapter: Exploring Identity Beyond Depression.
- Key elements: Rediscovering interests, goals, and strengths that may have been overshadowed by depression.
- Summary: Identity exploration helps reclaim your sense of self beyond the label of depression. Focusing on values, goals, and interests supports a vision for the future that includes growth, passion, and fulfilment.
- Ongoing practices: Periodically revisit personal goals and aspirations, setting intentions that align with your values. This reflective process keeps you motivated, helping you cultivate a life defined by purpose rather than symptoms.

10. Reframing Forgiveness and Letting Go

- Core chapter: Forgiveness and Letting Go
- Key elements: Releasing emotional burdens, practising forgiveness, reframing past experiences.
- Summary: Letting go of anger or resentment creates emotional freedom and supports healing. Forgiveness is a personal, self-compassionate act that allows space for peace

and growth.

- Ongoing practices: Practise forgiveness meditation, journal on forgiveness, and challenge unhelpful narratives. These practices help reduce stress and create space for emotional resilience.

11. Preventing Relapse with a Safety Net

- Core chapter: Understanding Relapse and Building a Safety Net.
- Key elements: Identifying early warning signs, building coping mechanisms, and reinforcing support systems.
- Summary: A relapse prevention plan anticipates challenges and prepares responses to maintain stability. Understanding personal triggers and maintaining a safety net builds preparedness and helps safeguard mental health.
- Ongoing practices: Regularly review and adapt your safety net, update coping strategies, and maintain open communication with your support network. Being proactive in prevention reduces the likelihood of relapse and supports long-term stability.

12. Embracing Positive Psychology and Personal Growth

- Core chapter: Gratitude, Kindness, and Positive Psychology.
- Key elements: Gratitude, kindness, strength, and personal growth.
- Summary: Positive psychology practices improve mental strength by focusing on gratitude, kindness, and personal strengths. These principles foster a positive, growth-oriented mindset that counteracts negative thought patterns.

- Ongoing practices: Continue daily gratitude, kindness exercises, and regularly set growth-focused goals. These practices reinforce a mindset that celebrates small victories and builds emotional strength.

A Roadmap for Lifelong Healing

As you move forward, remember that each layer of healing is interconnected. Here are steps to keep these principles alive:

- Regular self-check-ins: Schedule seasonal reflections on your physical, emotional, and mental health practices. Assess what's working, and make adjustments as needed.
- Set Intentional goals: Focus on one or two areas each season, whether that's deepening a spiritual practice, spending more time outdoors, or strengthening connections.
- Refresh and revisit: Return to specific chapters and practices in this book as you grow and encounter new challenges.
- Celebrate milestones: Take time to acknowledge your achievements, no matter how small. Celebrating your progress reinforces strength and supports long-term health.

Conclusion: Embracing Lifelong Resilience

Your recovery process is a testament to your strength and commitment to wellness. By layering each of these principles into your life, you create a comprehensive, adaptable approach to mental health that honours both your present needs and future growth. Embrace this journey as an evolving path, one that will carry you forward with strength, peace, and a deep connection to the life you're building.

References

Bratman, G. N., Hamilton, J. P., Hahn, K. S., Daily, G. C., & Gross, J. J. (2019). Nature experience reduces rumination and subgenual prefrontal cortex activation. Proceedings of the National Academy of Sciences, 112(28), 8567–8572.

Emmons, R. A., & Mishra, A. (2011). Why gratitude enhances well-being: What we know, what we need to know. In Sheldon, K. M., Kashdan, T. B., & Steger, M. F. (Eds.), Designing positive psychology: Taking stock and moving forward (pp. 248–262). Oxford University Press.

Goyal, M., Singh, S., Sibinga, E. M. S., Gould, N. F., Rowland-Seymour, A., Sharma, R., Berger, Z., Sleicher, D., Maron, D. D., Shihab, H. M., & Ranasinghe, P. D. (2014). Meditation programs for psychological stress and well-being: A systematic review and meta-analysis. JAMA Internal Medicine, 174(3), 357–368.

Koenig, H. G. (2012). Religion, spirituality, and health: The research and clinical implications. ISRN Psychiatry.

Ryff, C. D., & Singer, B. (2008). Know thyself and become what you are: A eudaimonic approach to psychological well-being. Journal of Happiness Studies, 9(1), 13–39.

Conclusion

As you reach the end of this book, take a moment to acknowledge the journey you've embarked on, a path that represents courage, persistence, and a commitment to self-care. Layered healing invites you to view your mental health recovery not as a destination but as a continually evolving path. Each chapter has offered tools, practices, and insights that build on one another, creating a framework you can carry forward and return to as you need.

This book is here for you to revisit whenever you need guidance or encouragement. Every layer you've explored – from building physical strength to cultivating emotional strength and finding connection – adds depth to the foundation you've built. You've seen firsthand that small, consistent steps create lasting change, and you've experienced how layered healing can help you reach your goal, whether that's remission, stability, or more profound health.

Moving Forward with Resilience and Self-Compassion

Life brings its own unique set of challenges, and recovery is often a winding road rather than a straight line. There may be times when you feel like you're moving forward and times when you feel you've slowed down. This is a natural part of healing, and each step – no matter how big or small – matters. The combined approach to healing gives you tools to manage life's inevitable ups and downs with self-compassion, helping you to meet each moment as it is.

As you move forward, remember to be gentle with yourself. Healing isn't about perfection; it's about progress, self-compassion, and resilience. Celebrate each milestone, however small, and honour the effort you put into every step. By caring for yourself in this way, you're not only nurturing your mental health but also building a life rooted in self-worth, strength, and purpose.

A Future That Holds Possibility

Layered healing doesn't just offer relief; it opens doors to new possibilities and allows you to imagine a future where you feel supported, strong, and connected. As you continue on this path, know that each layer you build contributes to something greater than the sum of its parts – a life that feels meaningful, fulfilling, and rich in connection.

Consider this journey an invitation to explore what brings you joy, fulfilment, and purpose. Whether that means reconnecting with old passions, nurturing relationships, or finding new avenues for growth, you now have the foundation to pursue these goals confidently. Healing is a way to reclaim your life, define it by hope and strength rather than by limitations, and recognise that you are worthy of all that lies ahead.

Final Words of Encouragement

Take each day as it comes, one layer at a time. Embrace the progress you make. However, it unfolds, and trust that each small step brings you closer to the life you envision. Healing isn't a linear path; it's a journey that grows with you, a journey that will continue to reveal its strength, beauty, and possibility as you move forward.

Let yourself celebrate each victory, no matter how small. Be patient with setbacks, and know that you are never alone on this path. The layers you've built – each practice, each insight, each step forward – will continue to support you, helping you rise with strength and move forward with hope.

You have the power to build the life you want, one layer at a time. May this journey bring you closer to the bright, fulfilling future you deserve.

Appendix: Key Studies Underpinning the Therapy Stack (Verified)

This appendix lists the core studies and reviews that support each layer. Entries have been checked and include the journal, year and a one-line summary.

Exercise & Movement

- Schuch FB, Vancampfort D, Richards J, Rosenbaum S, Ward PB, Stubbs B. "Exercise as a treatment for depression: a meta-analysis adjusting for publication bias." Journal of Psychiatric Research, 2016. Large antidepressant effect of exercise in RCTs.

- Cooney GM, Dwan K, Greig CA, et al. "Exercise for depression." Cochrane Database of Systematic Reviews, 2013; CD004366. Exercise reduces depressive symptoms versus control.

Nutrition & Diet

- Jacka FN, O'Neil A, Opie R, et al. "A randomised controlled trial of dietary improvement for adults with major depression (the SMILES trial)." BMC Medicine, 2017. 32.3% remission with dietary support vs 8.0% with social support at 12 weeks.

- Lassale C, Batty GD, Baghdadli A, et al. "Diet quality and depression risk: A systematic review and dose–response meta-analysis." Journal of Affective Disorders, 2018. Higher diet quality associated with lower depression risk.

Sleep

- Freeman D, Sheaves B, Goodwin GM, et al. "The effects of improving sleep on mental health (digital CBT for insomnia, OASIS trial)." The Lancet Psychiatry, 2017. Treating insomnia reduced depression and anxiety symptoms.

Mindfulness & MBCT

- Goyal M, Singh S, Sibinga EM, et al. "Meditation programs for psychological stress and health: a systematic review and meta-analysis." JAMA Internal Medicine, 2014. Small-to-moderate improvements in depression and anxiety.
- Kuyken W, Hayes R, Barrett B, et al. "PREVENT trial: MBCT vs maintenance antidepressants for preventing depressive relapse." The Lancet, 2015. MBCT performed similarly to maintenance antidepressants over 24 months.

Social Support & Connection

- Holt-Lunstad J, Smith TB, Layton JB. "Social relationships and mortality risk: a meta-analytic review." PLoS Medicine, 2010. Stronger social ties associated with ~50% higher survival odds.

- Cruwys T, Haslam SA, Dingle GA, et al. "Social group memberships protect against future depression, alleviate symptoms and prevent relapse." Social Science & Medicine, 2014. Joining groups linked with lower relapse risk.

Sunlight, Vitamin D & Light Therapy

- Bertone-Johnson ER, Powers SI, Spangler L, et al. "Vitamin D supplementation and depression in the Women's Health Initiative Calcium and Vitamin D Trial." American Journal of Epidemiology, 2012. No reduction in depression with 400 IU/day vitamin D3 + calcium.
- Pjrek E, Winkler D, Kasper S. "The Efficacy of Light Therapy in the Treatment of Seasonal Affective Disorder." Psychotherapy and Psychosomatics, 2019. Meta-analysis supports bright light therapy for SAD.

Therapies (CBT, ACT)

- Cuijpers P, Berking M, Andersson G, et al. "A meta-analysis of cognitive behavior therapy for adult depression, alone and in comparison with other treatments." Canadian Journal of Psychiatry, 2013. CBT shows moderate-to-large benefits vs control.
- A-Tjak JGL, Davis ML, Morina N, et al. "A meta-analysis of the efficacy of Acceptance and Commitment Therapy for clinically relevant mental and physical health problems." Psychotherapy and Psychosomatics, 2015. Small-to-moderate effects across conditions, including depression.

Relapse & Long-Term Outlook

- Hardeveld F, Spijker J, de Graaf R, Nolen WA, Beekman ATF. "Prevalence and predictors of recurrence of major depressive disorder in the adult population." Acta Psychiatrica Scandinavica, 2010. Recurrence common; previous episodes and residual symptoms key predictors.
- Piet J, Hougaard E. "The effect of mindfulness-based cognitive therapy for prevention of relapse in recurrent major depressive disorder: a systematic review and meta-analysis." Clinical Psychology Review, 2011. MBCT reduces relapse risk among recurrent depression.

References

Schuch, F. B., Vancampfort, D., Richards, J., Rosenbaum, S., Ward, P. B., & Stubbs, B. (2016). Exercise as a treatment for depression: A meta-analysis adjusting for publication bias. Journal of Psychiatric Research, 77, 42–51. https://doi.org/10.1016/j.jpsychires.2016.02.023

Cooney, G. M., Dwan, K., Greig, C. A., Lawlor, D. A., Rimer, J., Waugh, F. R., McMurdo, M., & Mead, G. E. (2013). Exercise for depression. Cochrane Database of Systematic Reviews, 9, CD004366. https://doi.org/10.1002/14651858.CD004366.pub6

Jacka, F. N., O'Neil, A., Opie, R., Itsiopoulos, C., Cotton, S., Mohebbi, M., … & Berk, M. (2017). A randomised controlled trial of dietary improvement for adults with major depression (the SMILES trial). BMC Medicine, 15, 23. https://doi.org/10.1186/s12916-017-0791-y

Lassale, C., Batty, G. D., Baghdadli, A., Jacka, F., Sánchez-Villegas, A., Kivimäki, M., & Akbaraly, T. (2018). Healthy dietary indices and risk of depressive outcomes: A systematic review and meta-analysis of observational studies. Molecular Psychiatry, 24, 965–986. https://doi.org/10.1038/s41380-018-0237-8

Freeman, D., Sheaves, B., Goodwin, G. M., Yu, L. M., Nickless, A., Harrison, P. J., … & Espie, C. A. (2017). The effects of improving sleep on mental health (OASIS): A randomised controlled trial with mediation analysis. The Lancet Psychiatry, 4(10), 749–758. https://doi.org/10.1016/S2215-0366(17)30328-0

Goyal, M., Singh, S., Sibinga, E. M. S., Gould, N. F., Rowland-Seymour, A., Sharma, R., … & Haythornthwaite, J. A. (2014). Meditation programs for psychological stress and health: A systematic review and meta-analysis. JAMA Internal Medicine, 174(3), 357–368. https://doi.org/10.1001/jamainternmed.2013.13018

Kuyken, W., Hayes, R., Barrett, B., Byng, R., Dalgleish, T., Kessler, D., … & Byford, S. (2015). Effectiveness of mindfulness-based cognitive therapy in prevention of depressive relapse (PREVENT): A randomised controlled trial. The Lancet, 386(9988), 63–73. https://doi.org/10.1016/S0140-6736(14)62222-4

Holt-Lunstad, J., Smith, T. B., & Layton, J. B. (2010). Social relationships and mortality risk: A meta-analytic review. PLoS Medicine, 7(7), e1000316. https://doi.org/10.1371/journal.pmed.1000316

Cruwys, T., Haslam, S. A., Dingle, G. A., Haslam, C., & Jetten, J. (2014). Depression and social identity: An integrative review. Personality and Social Psychology Review, 18(3), 215–238. https://doi.org/10.1177/1088868314523839

Bertone-Johnson, E. R., Powers, S. I., Spangler, L., Brunner, R. L., Michael, Y. L., Larson, J. C., ... & Wactawski-Wende, J. (2012). Vitamin D supplementation and depression in the Women's Health Initiative Calcium and Vitamin D Trial. American Journal of Epidemiology, 176(1), 1–13. https://doi.org/10.1093/aje/kwr482

Pjrek, E., Winkler, D., & Kasper, S. (2019). Bright light treatment in seasonal affective disorder. Psychotherapy and Psychosomatics, 88(3), 129–140. https://doi.org/10.1159/000500314

Cuijpers, P., Berking, M., Andersson, G., Quigley, L., Kleiboer, A., & Dobson, K. S. (2013). A meta-analysis of cognitive-behavioural therapy for adult depression, alone and in comparison with other treatments. Canadian Journal of Psychiatry, 58(7), 376–385. https://doi.org/10.1177/070674371305800702

A-Tjak, J. G. L., Davis, M. L., Morina, N., Powers, M. B., Smits, J. A. J., & Emmelkamp, P. M. G. (2015). A meta-analysis of the efficacy of acceptance and commitment therapy for clinically relevant mental and physical health problems. Psychotherapy and Psychosomatics, 84(1), 30–36. https://doi.org/10.1159/000365764

Hardeveld, F., Spijker, J., de Graaf, R., Nolen, W. A., & Beekman, A. T. F. (2010). Recurrence of major depressive disorder and its predictors in the general population: Results from the Netherlands Mental Health Survey and Incidence Study (NEMESIS). Acta Psychiatrica Scandinavica, 122(3), 184–191. https://doi.org/10.1111/j.1600-0447.2009.01519.x

Piet, J., & Hougaard, E. (2011). The effect of mindfulness-based cognitive therapy for prevention of relapse in recurrent major depressive disorder: A systematic review and meta-analysis. Clinical

Psychology Review, 31(6), 1032–1040. https://doi.org/10.1016/j.cpr.2011.05.002

Noetel, M., Sanders, T., Gallardo-Gómez, D., et al. (2024). Effect of exercise for depression: Systematic review and network meta-analysis of randomised controlled trials. BMJ, 384, e075847. https://doi.org/10.1136/bmj-2023-075847

Cochrane Collaboration. (2026). Exercise for depression in adults. Cochrane Database of Systematic Reviews.

Norwitz, N. G., Sethi, S., & Palmer, C. M. (2025). Ketogenic diet as a metabolic treatment for mental illness (KIND trial). Frontiers in Psychiatry, 16, 1396321.

Sethi, S., et al. (2026). Ketogenic diet vs phytochemical-rich control diet for treatment-resistant depression (DIME trial). JAMA Psychiatry.

Palmer, C. M., et al. (2026). Modified Delphi consensus on Ketogenic Metabolic Therapy (KMT) for serious mood disorders. Journal of Clinical Psychiatry.

Marschall, J., et al. (2025). A double-blind, placebo-controlled trial of psilocybin microdosing on subjective and behavioural measures. Neuropharmacology.

von Rotz, R., et al. (2024). Network meta-analysis of psilocybin-assisted therapy for depressive disorders. Psychological Medicine.

Therapeutic Goods Administration. (2023). Rescheduling of psilocybin and MDMA. Australian Government Department of Health and Aged Care.

Dray, J., et al. (2026). Social prescribing for youth mental health (Wellbeing While Waiting trial). The Lancet Child & Adolescent Health.

Nikolova, V. L., et al. (2025). Gut microbial diversity and depressive symptoms: A systematic review. Gut Microbiome.

Rucklidge, J. J., et al. (2025). Broad-spectrum micronutrients for antenatal depression (NUTRIMUM trial). University of Canterbury.

Caldieraro, M. A., et al. (2025). Photobiomodulation for depressive symptoms: A systematic review and meta-analysis. Journal of Affective Disorders, 348, 234–245.

Scott, A. J., Webb, T. L., Martyn-St James, M., Sherlock, G., & Rowse, G. (2024). Improving sleep quality leads to better mental health: A meta-analysis. Sleep Medicine Reviews, 60, 101556.

Chen, J., et al. (2026). Hyperbaric oxygen therapy for post-stroke depression: Clinical efficacy and neurobiological mechanisms. Frontiers in Neurology.

Index

Trauma 11, 12, 17, 21, 23, 28, 31
Trauma Releasing Exercises (TRE) 21, 23
Traumatic brain injury (TBI) 18

V

Vagus nerve 11, 15, 16, 21, 30

About the Author

Greg Doney is a mental health advocate with nearly 20 years of experience helping individuals recover from depression. Working alongside highly qualified professionals, Greg designs integrated recovery programs that combine evidence-based therapies with practical, compassionate guidance.

His work is grounded in a belief that lasting recovery comes from addressing the whole person — mind, body, and environment — and that the right combination of layered therapies can create meaningful, lasting change.

He is the author of Healing Trauma at the Cellular Level (2024) and Stacking Therapies for Depression Recovery (2026).